Digital Mammography

Digital Mammography

Physics and Instrumentation

Second Edition

Rob Davidson, PhD., MAppSc(MI), BBus, FASMIRT
University of Canberra
Bruce, Australia

Series Editor

Euclid Seeram, PhD., MSc., BSc., FCAMRT
Medical Imaging Advanced Studies
British Columbia Institute of Technology
Burnaby, British Columbia, Canada

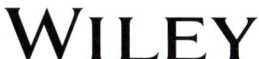

This edition first published 2026
© 2026 John Wiley & Sons Ltd

Edition History
John Wiley & Sons Ltd (1e, 2002)

The right of Rob Davidson to be identified as the author of this work has been asserted in accordance with law.

Registered Office(s)
John Wiley & Sons, Inc., 111 River Street, Hoboken, NJ 07030, USA
John Wiley & Sons Ltd, New Era House, 8 Oldlands Way, Bognor Regis, West Sussex, PO22 9NQ, UK

For details of our global editorial offices, customer services, and more information about Wiley products visit us at www.wiley.com.

The manufacturer's authorized representative according to the EU General Product Safety Regulation is Wiley-VCH GmbH, Boschstr. 12, 69469 Weinheim, Germany, e-mail: Product_Safety@wiley.com.

Wiley also publishes its books in a variety of electronic formats and by print-on-demand. Some content that appears in standard print versions of this book may not be available in other formats.

Limit of Liability/Disclaimer of Warranty
While the publisher and authors have used their best efforts in preparing this work, they make no representations or warranties with respect to the accuracy or completeness of the contents of this work and specifically disclaim all warranties, including without limitation any implied warranties of merchantability or fitness for a particular purpose. No warranty may be created or extended by sales representatives, written sales materials or promotional statements for this work. This work is sold with the understanding that the publisher is not engaged in rendering professional services. The advice and strategies contained herein may not be suitable for your situation. You should consult with a specialist where appropriate. The fact that an organization, website, or product is referred to in this work as a citation and/or potential source of further information does not mean that the publisher and authors endorse the information or services the organization, website, or product may provide or recommendations it may make. Further, readers should be aware that websites listed in this work may have changed or disappeared between when this work was written and when it is read. Neither the publisher nor authors shall be liable for any loss of profit or any other commercial damages, including but not limited to special, incidental, consequential, or other damages.

Library of Congress Cataloging-in-Publication Data Applied for:

Paperback ISBN: 9781119520818

Cover Design: Wiley
Cover Image: © andresr/Getty Images

Set in 11.5/13.5pt STIXTwoText by Straive, Pondicherry, India

Printed in Singapore
M091317230625

This book is dedicated to all mammographers/mammography technologists, mammography radiologists, and breast clinicians. Every day you help save lives of the 1 in 8 women in the world who will develop breast cancer and other breast diseases, yet most people do not know of your important role. On their behalf, I offer my sincere and grateful thanks.

Contents

Author Biography

Author:

Rob Davidson, PhD, MAppSc(MI), BBus, FASMIRT

Emeritus Professor, University of Canberra, Australia

Adjunct Research Professor, Fiji National University, Fiji

Professor Rob Davidson retired from the University of Canberra (UC) in February 2022 and was awarded the esteemed title of Emeritus Professor of the University of Canberra. In 2015, Professor Davidson developed and established the Medical Imaging and Ultrasound programs at UC. During Professor Davidson's appointment at UC, he was also the Head, School of Health Science and Discipline Lead, Medical Radiation Sciences. Rob is also an Adjunct Research Professor in Medical Imaging, College of Medicine, Nursing & Health Sciences at Fiji National University and has held an adjunct appointment at RMIT University.

Rob was the second person to be appointed as a Full Professor in Medical Imaging/Medical Radiation Sciences in Australia. He has previously held roles as a Professor at Charles Sturt University (CSU), Associate Professor at RMIT University and at Curtin University, and Senior Lecturer at CSU. Prior to becoming an academic, Rob was employed as a Medical Imaging Clinician for approximately 10 years, followed by a further 9 years in sales/marketing roles.

In 2003, Rob completed his Master's in Medical Imaging; in 2006, he received his PhD in Medical Imaging/Physics; and in 2008, he gained Fellowship of the Australian Society for Medical Imaging and Radiation Therapy (ASMIRT). Early in his academic career, he was awarded the 2001 UniServe Science National Science Teaching Award as the best university science lecturer in Australia.

Rob has been the Editor-in-Chief of *The Radiographer*, the then journal of the Australian Institute of Radiographer/ASMIRT; was Deputy Editor of the Canadian journal, *Journal of Medical Imaging and Radiation Sciences;* and is currently on the Board of the *Journal of Medical Radiation Sciences.*

Rob's research focus is on dose/image quality in mammography, planar radiography, and CT; digital image processing in medical imaging; and is currently part of an international team looking at new imaging methods for the improved detection of prostate cancer. He has been a chief investigator on multiple research grants, has over 70 peer-reviewed publications, authored/coauthored six book chapters. Rob has also been the keynote speaker at multiple international conferences, supervised/cosupervised approximately 20 PhD and Master's by research students, and examined multiple higher degree by research theses. Professor Davidson has established international research colleagues in the United States, Canada, Kuwait, Fiji, Saudi Arabia, The Netherlands, and Taiwan. PhD students have come to Australia to be supervised by Rob from Singapore, China, Saudi Arabia, and Fiji.

Contributor

Liz Bowey, CCPM, ABIC, GCertMR (Breast Ultrasound)

Retired Mammographer/Breast Sonographer

Liz, after graduating in 1973 from the then South Australian Institute of Technology, now UniSA, worked in several places in various states of Australia. Once she moved back to Adelaide, her interest in mammography grew. Liz worked for Dr Jones & Partners, now Jones Radiology, which placed a high value and gave support for top-level breast imaging. Liz earned her first Certificate of Clinical Proficiency in Mammography (CCPM) in 1997, which she kept renewed until her retirement. In 1998–1999, Liz studied for and attained the Graduate Certificate in Medical Imaging (Breast Ultrasound), the first person in the Jones Radiology to achieve this qualification. Liz was part of a team that helped set up the Breast Centre of Excellence at Burnside Hospital, where the X-ray department worked closely with a team of breast surgeons and pathologists. In 2001, Liz was appointed Chief of Mammography. Her role included setting up a mammography training program; organizing and supervising basic and advanced training for staff; organizing attendance at BreastScreen SA (BSSA) training programs/ conferences; organizing site accreditation for the Australian/ New Zealand RANZCR MQAP standards; QA/QC program; CPD programs; purchasing new equipment; liaising with referrers; giving presentations to staff at BSSA professional development days and also to referrers; and serving as guest lecturer for breast ultrasound at UniSA. In 2005, Liz was awarded the Advanced Breast Imaging Certificate (ABIC) by the Australian Institute of Radiography (AIR), now the Australian Society for Medical Imaging and Radiation Therapy (ASMIRT).

Liz also worked concurrently for BreastScreen SA on a casual basis for about 12 years in the assessment clinics, doing breast ultrasound, biopsies, etc. This work gave her a valuable insight into the workings of BreastScreen and was helpful in her role in Jones Radiology.

Liz retired from radiography in 2017. She was very proud of what was achieved in her time at Jones Radiology and BSSA. At these organizations, she worked with many dedicated and caring staff to ensure the standard of mammography remained high, giving a great service to their clients.

Series Editor's Foreword

Wiley's *Rad Tech's Guides Series* in radiologic technology is intended to provide clear and comprehensive coverage of a wide range of topics and prepare students to write their entry-to-practice registration examination. Additionally, this series can be used by working technologists to review essential and practical concepts and principles and to use them as tools to enhance their daily skills during the examination of patients in the radiology department.

The *Rad Tech's Guides Series* features short books covering the fundamental core curriculum topics for radiologic technologists at both the diploma and the specialty levels, as well as acting as knowledge sources for continuing education as defined by the American Registry for Radiologic Technologists (ARRT).

Titles in the series include books on radiologic physics, equipment operation, patient care, radiographic technique, radiologic procedures, radiation protection, image production and evaluation, and quality control. You may have noticed that this book lacks the Rad Tech's Guides title on the front cover. Thematically and structurally, this is very much a Rad Tech's Guide, but we felt that the readership extended beyond radiologic technologists and made the decision to broaden the scope by removing the series title.

In *Digital Mammography: Physics and Instrumentation*, Dr. Rob Davidson, a renowned educator and expert in radiologic sciences and technology from the University of Canberra and other universities in Australia, presents clear and concise coverage of the physics and instrumentation of digital mammography. More details of his academic activities are provided in his biography included in this book. He has coauthored Chapter 1 with Liz Bowey, CCPM, ABIC, G Cert MR (Breast Ultrasound), and her biography is also listed in this book.

Topics include why mammography? Fundamental physics of mammography, equipment components, image quality, dose consideration, digital breast tomosynthesis, quality control issues of primary significance to quality mammography, and finally artificial intelligence in mammography.

Dr. Davidson has done an excellent job in explaining significant concepts that are mandatory for the successful performance of quality digital mammography in clinical practice. Students, technologists, clinicians, and educators alike will find this book a worthwhile addition to their libraries.

Enjoy the pages that follow; remember, your patients will benefit from your wisdom.

Euclid Seeram, PhD, MSc. BSc, FCAMRT
Series Editor
British Columbia, Canada

Acknowledgments

First, I thank the author of the first edition of this textbook, Donald R. Jacobson, PhD, DABMP, who has provided an excellent template for this second edition. His knowledge of mammography physics and instrumentation, which shone through in that text, I am sure has guided many potential and current clinical people in the breast imaging field of the medical radiation sciences.

Next, my thanks go to Euclid Seeram, PhD, MSc, BSc, FCAMRT, for inviting me to revise and update Donald's textbook. Euclid is a great colleague and friend, and I have had the privilege to be a part of his supervising team for his PhD candidature; we have undertaken research together and have coauthored chapters and a book. Euclid, you are a great mate.

Importantly, thank you to the people who have allowed me to use their images in this book. We all belong to the medical imaging community, and I think the old adage of "an image says a thousand words" is an understatement in our field. By providing these images, you have saved the readers much time.

I also thank Liz Bowey, my sister, for writing the clinical part of Chapter 1. Liz and I belong to a medical family, and as such, I think our career directions were easy to choose. Liz has been a dedicated mammography/breast sonographer for many years, and I am sure her patients have benefited from her clinical skills and calming manner. Thanks, sis!

Finally, I thank Debbie and the rest of my family for giving me the time to focus on writing this textbook. You all have supported and encouraged me in doing this when I could have spent more time with you.

1 Why Mammography?

Why Mammography? The Clinical Reasons, by Liz Bowey

When first considering the topic of "Why mammography?", any instinctive reaction should be "Why not?" Mammography can be used as a screening tool in asymptomatic women, or as a diagnostic tool to investigate lumps or changes to the breast. In both cases, it is a really important part of caring for women's health and well-being. Mammography is currently the best way to discover early breast cancers. It can detect breast cancer before it shows physical symptoms. Mammograms have also been proven to reduce the risk of dying from breast cancer which affects up to one in eight women in their lifetime. Early detection of cancers and precancerous lesions has increased with continual improvements in mammography. Early detection/early diagnosis is still the best way of ensuring a good outcome, so why would we not make use of mammography?

Most women in developed countries have access to free screening mammography. Those who have symptoms that

Digital Mammography: Physics and Instrumentation, Second Edition.
Rob Davidson.
© 2026 John Wiley & Sons Ltd. Published 2026 by John Wiley & Sons Ltd.

need close follow-up, or are following up on a suspicious area, will need diagnostic mammography which is often accompanied by breast ultrasound and other breast image modalities as needed to assist in making the diagnosis. The mammogram, whether screening or diagnostic, is a low-dose X-ray examination, and both use the same type of equipment and require well-trained staff.

Good mammography is a combination of many things. Digital mammographic image examples are shown in Figure 1.1. Having access to state-of-the-art equipment is paramount. The importance of this will be covered in the rest of this book. Well-trained mammographers and radiologists are the other essential requirements to produce good mammography. A good

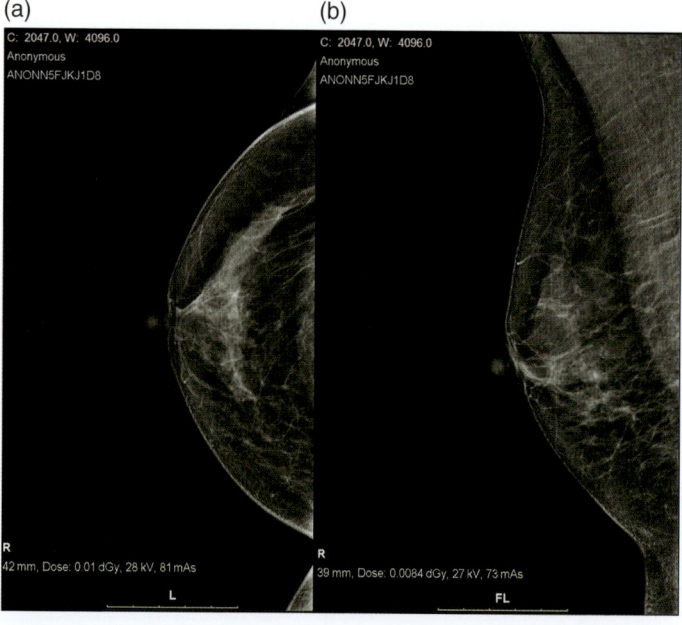

Figure 1.1 An example of a digital mammographic examination of the right breast. (a) A cranio-caudal view *and* (b) a mediolateral oblique view. *Source:* With permission of BreastScreen ACT, Canberra, Australia.

mammographer/mammography technologist will put the client at ease. This is essential as it is easier to position a breast and get really good coverage if the client is relaxed. Getting a few more millimeters of breast tissue into the field of view can mean seeing a cancer that may have been missed. It is a real skill to achieve the best positioning possible for each client. Breast shape and size, body habitus, and client maneuverability are just a few of the issues to deal with. The procedure is also much less uncomfortable for the relaxed client than a tense one!

Why Digital Mammography? An Overview of the Technical Reasons, by Rob Davidson

Currently, planar X-ray imaging, including mammography and general X-ray imaging, uses digital radiography (DR) recording methods. DR imaging requires the anatomy of interest to have differing amounts of X-ray attenuation, also known as subject contrast, so the X-ray exit intensities from those anatomical regions differ by at least 5%. In general X-ray DR imaging, anatomical regions, for example, of the chest and bones, the attenuation difference in that anatomical region is significantly greater than 5%. If the attenuation differences are less than 5%, the detectors will not be able to detect differences in the X-ray beam's exit intensities and there will be no differences in gray levels and image contrast in the displayed image.

One of the main advantages of computed tomography, arguably the main advantage, is CT's low contrast resolution of around 0.25%. In other words, there needs to be an anatomical subject contrast of greater than 0.25%. The advantage of this is seen in CT imaging of the brain and abdomen, where general planar X-ray imaging cannot visualize gray matter/white matter differences and has difficulty in visualizing different abdominal organs.

The breast tissue is composed of fibroglandular, adipose, blood vessel, and ductal tissues. These tissues and breast cancers have very similar X-ray attenuation characteristics. Figure 1.2 shows a plot of linear attenuation of fibroglandular, adipose, and cancer tissues. Linear attenuation coefficients of all matter decrease in differences as X-ray photon energies are increased. General planar X-ray imaging typically has its lowest peak voltage, kVp, setting at 40 kVp; however, higher kVp settings are generally used. Mammography X-ray imaging units have lower kVp settings and hence lower X-ray photon energies can predominate in the X-ray beam. Using lower X-ray photon energies, breast tissues have greater X-ray attenuation difference and breast cancers can be visualized from healthy breast tissues.

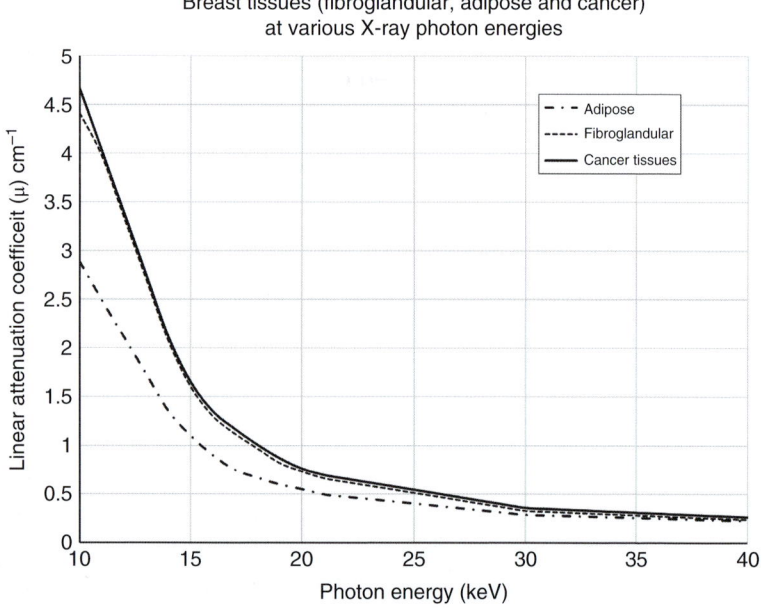

Figure 1.2 A plot of linear attenuation coefficients of breast fibroglandular, adipose, and cancer tissues at various photon energies (keV).
Source: Adapted from Hubbell and Seltzer (2004), and Soares, Gobo et al. (2020).

Mammography X-ray tubes' target and filtration material are also designed to optimize the X-ray photon spectrum and energies. General X-ray tubes typically have tungsten targets, primarily to maximize X-ray photon production, and aluminum filters, primarily to reduce the number of low-energy X-ray photons reaching the patient that would increase the radiation dose to the patient. Such general X-ray tubes are not designed nor optimized for imaging anatomy with a low inherent subject contrast.

X-ray image contrast is partially dependent on the thickness of the object being imaged. Image contrast is reduced and image quality is degraded when X-ray photons are scattered by the object and reach the image detector. The greater the object thickness, the greater the amount of scattered radiation. Compression is used to reduce breast thickness and improve image contrast and hence able to visualize greater differences between cancers and normal breast tissue. Compression in general X-ray imaging is rarely used clinically.

An X-ray image's spatial resolution, the ability to record and display detail in the image is primarily dependent on both the spatial details of the detector and the size of the focal spot where the X-ray photons are produced. The smaller the detector's pixel size and the smaller the focal spot, the greater the spatial resolution of the system. Breast imaging needs to be able to detect very small objects such as mammary microcalcifications (MCs). The presence of MCs can indicate premalignant and malignant breast lesions. General X-ray unit detectors typically have pixel sizes between 120 and 160 μm, whereas mammography unit pixel sizes are typically between 70 and 100 μm. The X-ray tube focal spot is much smaller in mammography units compared to general X-ray units. Typically, in a mammography unit, the focal spot sizes are: the small focal spot is around 0.10–0.15 mm, and the large focal spot is around 0.3 mm. Common general X-ray tube focal spot sizes are: the small focal spot is 0.6 mm, and the large focal spot is around 1.2 mm.

With small focal spot sizes, the X-ray tube filament current is much less than the current used in general X-ray tubes. Typical mammography filament currents are: 10–50 milliamps (mA) used for the small focal spot and 100–200 mA for the large focal spot. Large focal spot currents in general imaging can be 1,000–2,000 mA and even higher for angiography units. The time of the X-ray exposure is dependent on the mA being used and on the distance of the source of X-rays, the source-to-image distance (SID). To keep exposure times in mammography shorter, the SID is reduced compared to typical SIDs of 100 cm in general X-ray imaging.

An X-ray beam diverges as it travels from the focal point. The central ray of an X-ray beam is usually aligned so it will be at a right angle to the center of the detector/image plate. If this approach was used in mammography, the breast tissue near the chest wall furthest from the image plate would not be in the X-ray beam and as such, not imaged, potentially missing pathology. Mammography X-ray units' designs are to angle and align the X-ray tube so that the X-ray beam is at a right angle to the edge of the image plate that is closest to the patient's chest wall. This approach in mammography units allows the beam to skim the chest wall and include the maximum amount of breast tissue in the image.

Other X-ray mammography technologies that require digital techniques have been developed. These are digital breast tomosynthesis (DBT) and contrast-enhanced digital mammography (CEDM).

These mammography characteristics discussed earlier have been developed over many years. Prior to 1969, general X-ray units with tungsten targets and X-ray film were used for breast imaging. Mammography unit development has made many changes since the 1960s and the main ones are given in Table 1.1.

The following chapters will discuss in more detail the physics and instrumentation requirements in digital mammography to create images that assist in the diagnosis of breast cancer and other breast diseases.

Table 1.1 X-ray Mammography Unit Development Timetable.

Year	Development
1969	Dedicated mammography unit with molybdenum target and compression
1971	Xerography mammography unit
1972	Dedicated mammography film-screen systems
1977	Micro-focal spot sizes for magnification mammography
1978	Mammography grids
2000	Digital mammography unit
2011	Digital breast tomosynthesis (DBT) and contrast-enhanced digital mammography (CEDM)

Bibliography

Diffey, J. L. (2015). "A comparison of digital mammography detectors and emerging technology." *Radiography* 21(4): 315–323.

Fredenberg, E., Willsher, P., Moa, E., Dance, D. R., Young, K. C. and Wallis, M. G. (2018). "Measurement of breast-tissue x-ray attenuation by spectral imaging: fresh and fixed normal and malignant tissue." *Physics in Medicine & Biology* 63(23): 235003.

Haus, A. G. (2002). "Historical technical developments in mammography." *Technology in Cancer Research & Treatment* 1(2): 119–126.

Hubbell, J. and Seltzer, S. (2004). X-ray mass attenuation coefficients, NIST Standard Reference Database 126. Technology, N. I. o. S. a.

Kalaf, J. M. (2014). "Mammography: a history of success and scientific enthusiasm." *Radiologia Brasileira* 47(4): Vii-viii.

Logullo, A. F., Prigenzi, K. C. K., Nimir, C., Franco, A. F. V. and Campos, M. (2022). "Breast microcalcifications: past, present and future (Review)." *Molecular and Clinical Oncology* 16(4): 81.

Nicosia, L., Gnocchi, G., Gorini, I., Venturini, M., Fontana, F., Pesapane, F., Abiuso, I., Bozzini, A. C., Pizzamiglio, M., Latronico, A., Abbate, F., Meneghetti, L., Battaglia, O., Pellegrino, G. and Cassano, E. (2023). "History of mammography: analysis of breast imaging diagnostic achievements over the last century." *Healthcare* 11(11): 1596.

Soares, L. D. H., Gobo, M. S. S. and Poletti, M. E. (2020). "Measurement of the linear attenuation coefficient of breast tissues using polienergetic x-ray for energies from 12 to 50 keV and a silicon dispersive detector." *Radiation Physics and Chemistry* 167: 108226.

Tomal, A., Mazarro, I., Kakuno, E. M. and Poletti, M. E. (2010). "Experimental determination of linear attenuation coefficient of normal, benign and malignant breast tissues." *Radiation Measurements* 45(9): 1055–1059.

2 Mammographic Instrumentation and Physics

Chapter at a Glance

- Introduction
- Instrumentation
- X-ray Generator
- Mammography Unit Geometry
- X-ray Tube, Target, and Filter Materials
- X-ray Production
- Magnification
- Bibliography

Introduction

Chapter 1 discussed the reasons, both clinical and technical, for the need for mammography and the specialized equipment that is used. This chapter will look at mammography principles and the technical aspects of that equipment in more detail. The details provided assume a basic understanding of general X-ray equipment and principles and will focus on the differences between general X-ray and mammography equipment and physical principles.

Digital Mammography: Physics and Instrumentation, Second Edition.
Rob Davidson.
© 2026 John Wiley & Sons Ltd. Published 2026 by John Wiley & Sons Ltd.

Producing quality mammograms involves five essential steps. These steps are:

1. X-ray production
2. X-ray interaction with matter, in this case, breast tissue
3. Capturing and recording transmitted X-rays
4. Digital image processing of the recorded image
5. Displaying and viewing the image

Figure 2.1 shows a representation of these steps. The quality of the final image depends on the integrity of each step, a weakness in any one step will reduce the quality of the final image and the ability of clinicians to make an accurate diagnosis. Imaging specialists must understand these steps so that any loss of image quality can be related back to the appropriate step. This chapter will focus on the first two points stated earlier and Chapter 3 will focus on the last three points.

Instrumentation

X-ray equipment or instrumentation used in mammography, in principle, is very similar to general planar X-ray equipment. However, there are some significant differences. The instrumentation needed in both are:

- a high-voltage generator, to produce a high voltage that is applied across the X-ray tube. The mammography high-voltage generator only differs from a general high-voltage generator in that the maximum voltage, the current in the X-ray tube, and as such the X-ray tube output is less.
- an X-ray tube, to produce the X-ray beam. There are significant differences between mammography and general X-ray tubes.
- an image plate/detector, to capture the transmitted X-ray photons. There are differences between mammography

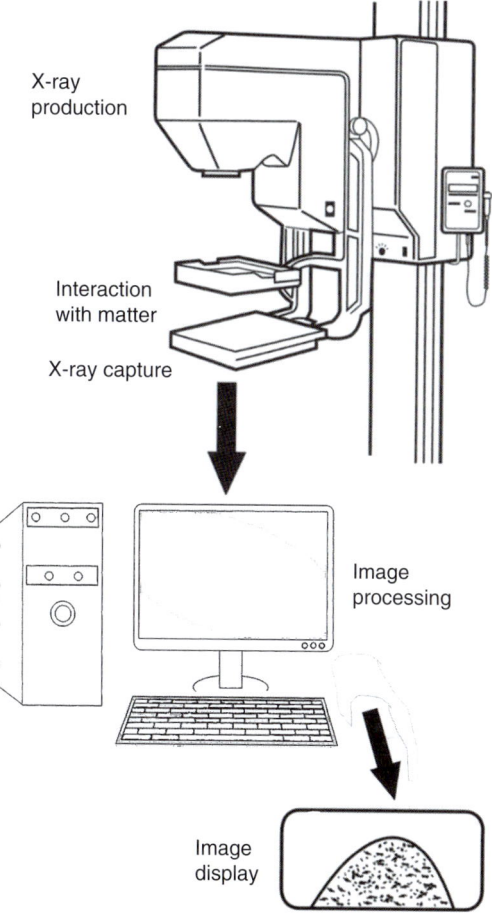

X-ray
production

Interaction
with matter

X-ray capture

Image
processing

Image
display

Figure 2.1 The five essential steps in producing quality mammograms.

and general X-ray image plates/detectors. The X-ray tube and image plate have a fixed relationship between them and the support arm of the X-ray tube, which in tomosynthesis units can move in an arc.

■ computer and display screen.

In mammography, several other things are different and one of the main ones is a compression paddle that is used to reduce breast thickness. Compression is very rarely in general planar X-ray imaging.

A diagram of a mammography unit, showing the relationships between the X-ray tube, the beam itself, the compression paddle, the breast being imaged, the X-ray grid, and the image plate/receptors/detectors, is shown in Figure 2.2.

The image plate/flat panel detector, computer, and display screen will be discussed in Chapter 3.

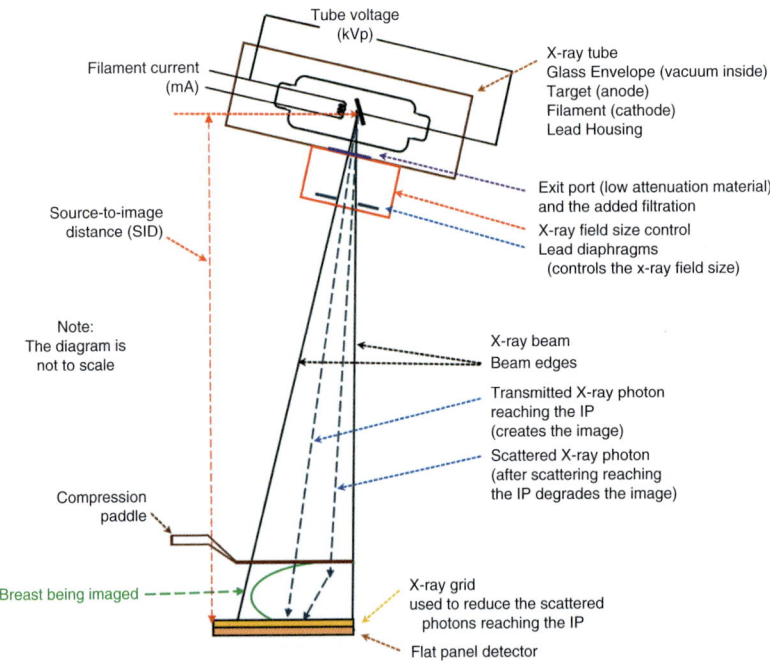

Figure 2.2 Diagram of a mammography unit showing the relationship among the instrumentation, the X-ray beam, and the breast being imaged.

X-ray Generator

The mammography X-ray tube and other general X-ray tubes require two power supplies, which together are referred to as the X-ray generator.

- Filament heating power supply:
  The filament temperature determines the number of electrons emitted, thus the tube current (mA) and the quantity of X-rays. A hotter filament, controlled by the filament current, emits more electrons. Typical values are around 10 V and 5 A (50 W).
- High-voltage power supply:
  The line or incoming voltage is transformed into higher voltages needed in X-ray production. The typical range used in mammography is 20–30,000 V, that is, 20–30 peak kilovolts (kVp), though some mammography X-ray units have higher voltages. The typical maximum power of a generator would be 35 kVp × 200 mA = 7,000 W (7.0 kW). The kVp determines the energy of the electrons bombarding the target and is therefore one of the factors, along with target and filter material, that subsequently determine the energy of the X-ray photons produced and reaching the breast.

High-Frequency Generator Technology

High-frequency X-ray generators have been in use since the 'mid-1980s and mammography units were the first to use this technology. Prior to high-frequency technology, single- and three-phase generators were used. In single-phase generators, the voltage varied between zero (0) volts and the set kVp. This is shown in Figure 2.3a which shows a full-rectified (no voltage below zero) waveform. The issue is that during one phase or cycle (one 50th or one 60th of a second depending on the country's power supply), the voltage applied across the X-ray to generate the X-ray varies from zero, with no X-ray photon being generated; to varying voltages below the set maximum voltage to for a few milliseconds; to the desired set maximum voltage, that is, the set kVp. Such a high-voltage waveform provides mainly low-energy photons that contribute little to the image and increase patient dose significantly. This single-phase waveform was improved upon with the development of three-phase generators with 6- or 12-phase rectifiers, the resultant waveform is shown in Figure 2.3b. The voltage across the X-ray tube varies less over a cycle.

High-frequency X-ray generators further reduce the voltage ripple and as such, the voltage during a cycle remains closer to the set kVp. The high-frequency waveform is shown in Figure 2.3c. As a result of using this waveform, the X-ray photon energies vary less during a cycle.

The voltage ripple, the amount of voltage variation during a cycle, for all generator types is defined as

$$\text{voltage ripple} = \frac{\text{maximum voltage} - \text{minimum voltage}}{\text{maximum voltage}} \times 100\%$$

Table 2.1 shows the voltage ripple for various waveforms.

Some benefits of high-frequency generator technology are as follows:

- smaller and lighter generator (more compact)
- more constant output voltage (less voltage ripple)
- reduced patient dose due to the reduced variation of the voltage
- repeatable and accurate X-ray technique delivery
- closed-loop feedback

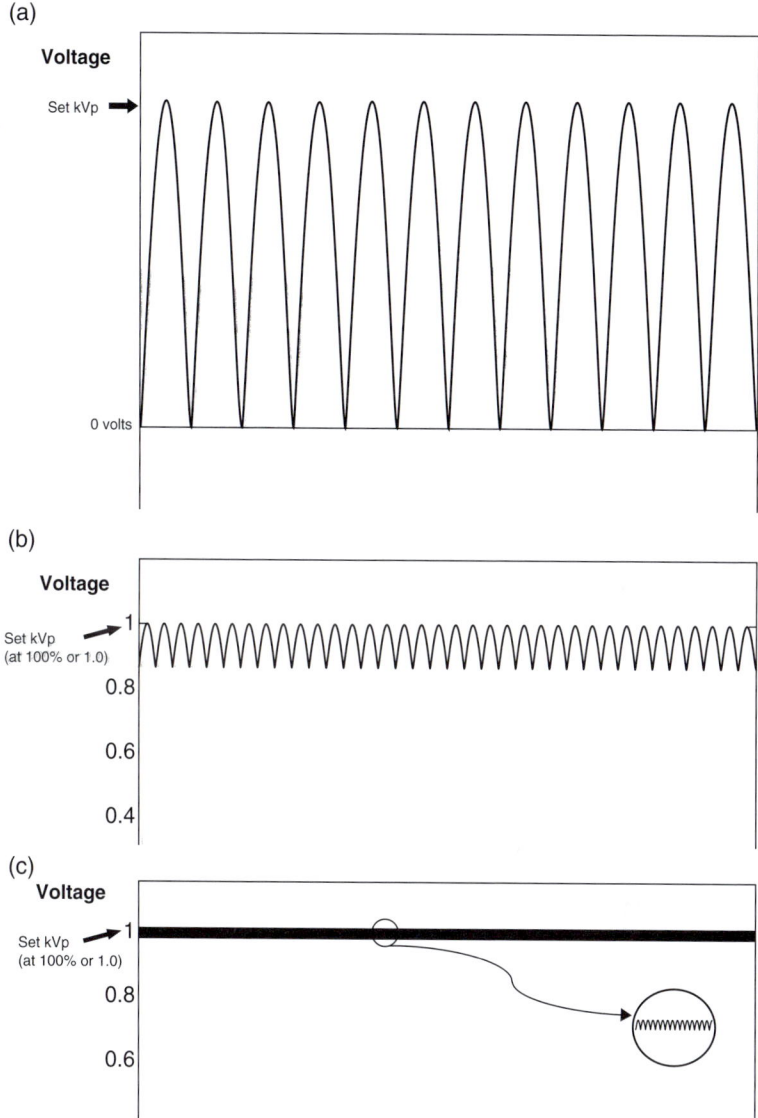

Figure 2.3 (a) Single-phase voltage waveform over a number of 50/60 Hz cycles showing the voltage applied across the X-ray tube varying from 0 V to the set kVp. Note that no voltage is negative. (b) Three-phase voltage waveform showing the voltage applied across the X-ray tube varying from approximately 85% of the set kVp to the set kVp. (c) A high-frequency voltage waveform showing the voltage applied across the X-ray tube varying from approximately 97% of the set kVp to the set kVp, with the inset showing the high-frequency ripple.

Table 2.1 Voltage Ripple of Various X-ray Generator Waveforms.

Waveform	Voltage Ripple
1Φ (50/60 Hz)	100%
3Φ (6 pulse, 150/180 Hz)	13–25%
3Φ (12 pulse, 300/440 Hz)	7–10%
High frequency (10–100 kHz)	<5%

- generator monitors the output voltage
- feedback from the output to the input of the high-voltage transformer
- produces more constant output energy (kVp)
- filament heating current is also regulated by mA feedback, which produces a more consistent tube current (mA)

Mammography X-ray Tube, Filter, and Collimator

An X-ray tube is an example of an electronic device known as a diode as it contains two electrodes – the negative cathode, the filament, and the positive anode, the target. A diagram of the X-ray tube is shown in Figure 2.4.

Electrons produced at the cathode are accelerated by the high positive voltage of the anode where they interact with the anode material to produce X-rays. The X-ray tube contains a vacuum, and as such the projectile electrons travel to the target without colliding with air molecules. When they reach the target, the electrons typically travel at approximately half the speed of light (approximately 150,000 km per second or 93,000 miles per second).

Cathode: In most mammography tubes, the cathode contains two tungsten–thorium filaments, one for the large focal

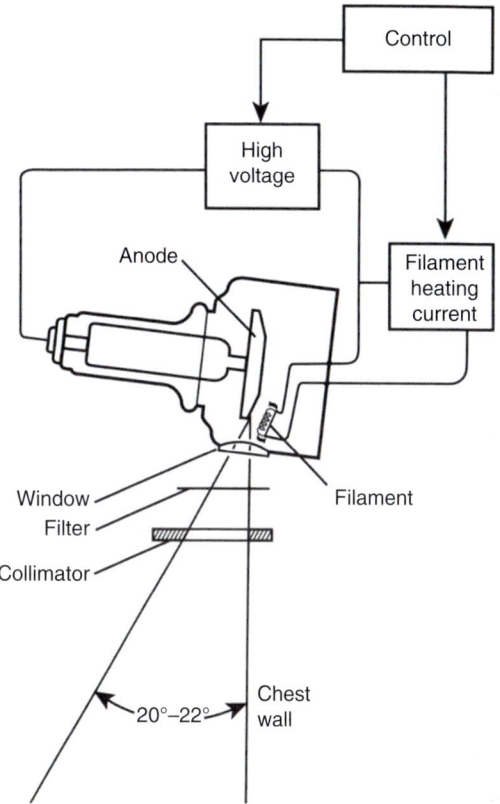

Figure 2.4 Diagrammatic representation of a mammography X-ray tube showing internal tube components and the filter and collimator. Also note the vertical beam along the chest wall.

spot and one for the small focal spot. As an electrical current passes through the filament, the filament becomes white hot due to the resistance in the filament wire. Electrons are then thermionically emitted, the so-called boiled-off, and when the voltage is applied across the X-ray tube, the thermionically emitted electrons are attracted to the positive anode, the target. The emitted electrons become the tube current, which is measured in milliamperes (mA). Some properties of the cathode are the following:

- The filament for the large focal spot, which typically has a stated size of 0.3 mm, usually operates at a maximum of 200 mA tube current, although this varies between manufacturers.
- Tube current is often limited at high or low kilovolts peak (kVp).
  - At high kVp, the limit is from the target's-heating limitations
  - At low kVp, the limit is from space-charge limitations, which is a phenomenon that limits the number of thermionically emitted electrons due to their own negative electrostatic charge reducing the amount of thermionically emitted electrons.
- The filament for the small focal spot (typically 0.1–0.15 mm) operates at 25–35 mA tube current.

The small filaments and hence small focal spot sizes used in mammography X-ray tubes are dictated by the need in mammography for high spatial resolution imaging. Note that both the mammography large and small focal spots are smaller than those used in general X-rays. However, these small filaments can only have low tube currents compared to general X-ray tubes. As such, the number of photons produced in a given amount of time will also be reduced.

The orientation of the cathode, either toward or away from the patient's chest wall, is shown in Figure 2.5. The advantages and disadvantages of each orientation are discussed in detail later.

The filaments in all X-ray tubes are placed inside a focusing cup. The purpose of the focusing cup is to reduce the spread of the electrons as they travel toward the anode/target. In mammography X-ray tubes, the focusing cup is biased. This means that there is a small negative charge on the cup, compared to

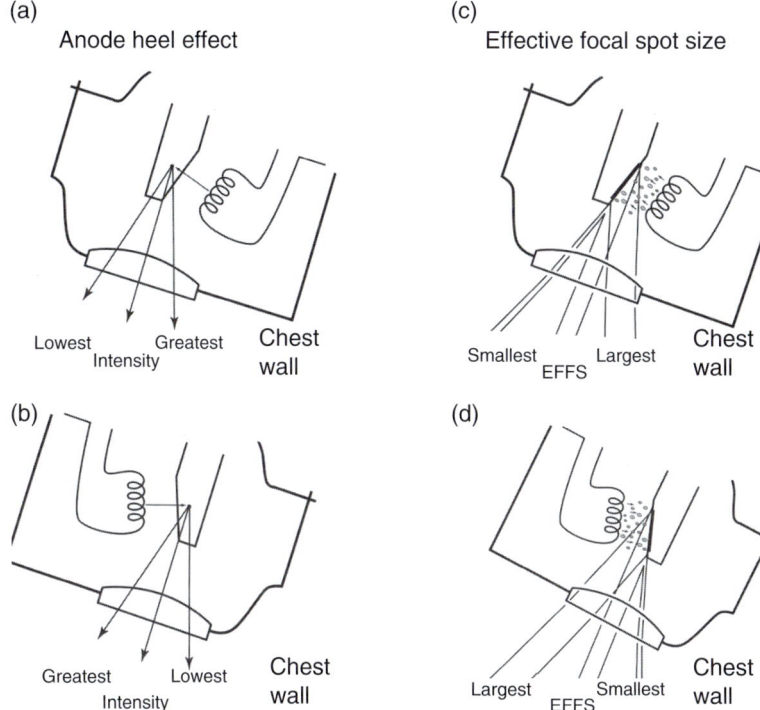

Figure 2.5 Orientation of the cathode and anode in the X-ray tube to the patient's chest wall. (a) and (c) show the cathode nearest the chest wall and (b) and (d) show the cathode away from the chest wall. The advantages and disadvantages are discussed in the text.

the cup being grounded or at zero volts, which is the method used in general X-rays. The negative bias approach better focuses on the electrons as they travel through the electrical field from the cup and onto the anode. An additional advantage of this is that engineers can regularly check the focal spot size, that is, where the electrons strike the target, and, if needed can adjust the power supply to increase the negative bias bringing the focal spot size back into the desired specifications. Figure 2.6a shows a diagrammatic representation of a general X-ray tube focusing

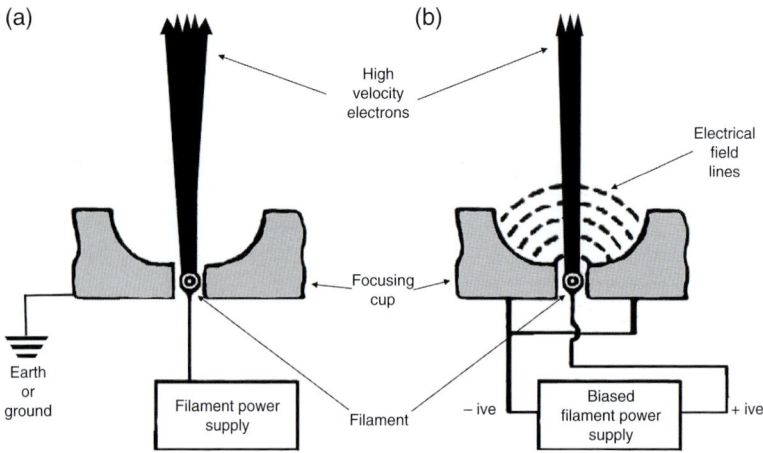

Figure 2.6 (a) A conventional X-ray tube focusing cup and (b) a mammography-biased focusing cup.

cup and in Figure 2.6b a mammography-biased focusing cup with the resultant reduced spread of the electron beam.

Anode: The positive electrode of the X-ray tube is the anode. The kinetic energy of the high-velocity electrons is converted into X-ray energy in a thin layer of the surface of the anode, which is referred to as the target.

- All modern mammographic tubes have a rotating anode. A typical anode diameter is 10 cm or 4 in., and as such the area of the focal track is approximately 300 times larger than the area of the actual focal spot. This allows the heat produced by the high-velocity electrons to be dissipated over a larger area than if using a stationary anode.
- The typical anode heat capacity is 300,000 heat units (HU) or greater.
- The target materials are typically molybdenum (Mo), rhodium (Rh), or tungsten (W). Mammography units typically have more than one target material.

Focal spot: The point on the anode where the high-velocity electron strikes the anode is called the target or focal spot. As discussed earlier, there are usually two cathode filaments so there are two focal spots of differing sizes, a small and large focal spot. The line focus principle is used to show the effective focal spot size. The filament size, and hence electron beam size, and the anode angle dictate the size of the area where the electrons strike the target, the actual focal spot size. What is important is the effective focal spot size, which is discussed in detail later. Common effective focal spot sizes are 0.1–0.15 mm for the small focal spot and 0.3 mm for the large focal spot. Note that all actual and effective focal spots are an area with two dimensions.

The International Electrotechnical Commission (IEC) has set specifications, IEC60336, for tolerances of focal spot size. In mammography, these are shown in Table 2.2.

X-ray production: Basically, in an X-ray tube, X-ray photons are produced when high-velocity electrons with high kinetic energy are slowed or stopped giving up their kinetic energy as electromagnetic (EM) energy. EM radiation has both wave and

Table 2.2 International Electrotechnical Commission (IEC) Focal Spot Tolerances (from IEC60336: 2005 and the US Mammography Quality Standards Act [MQSA]).

Nominal Focal Spot Size (mm)	Maximum Focal Spot Dimension (mm)	
	Width (mm)	Length (mm)
0.10	0.15	0.15
0.15	0.23	0.23
0.20	0.30	0.30
0.25	0.38	0.38
0.30	0.45	0.65
0.40	0.60	0.85

particle (called photons or quanta) properties – more on this in Chapter 6. X-ray production occurs in two situations, which are

- Bremsstrahlung (from German meaning braking radiation) interactions: If a high-velocity electron passes in close proximity to the positively charged nucleus of the atom, electrostatic forces between them cause the electron to change direction. The closer the electron is to the nucleus, the greater the change of direction and the greater the amount of energy is given off. If the electron strikes the nucleus, all of its kinetic energy is converted to EM radiation. Only a few electrons will strike the nucleus of the atom, more will pass close to the nucleus and even more at increasing distance from the nucleus. X-ray photons produced by Bremsstrahlung interactions are shown and plotted as a straight line (without attenuation) in Figure 2.7.

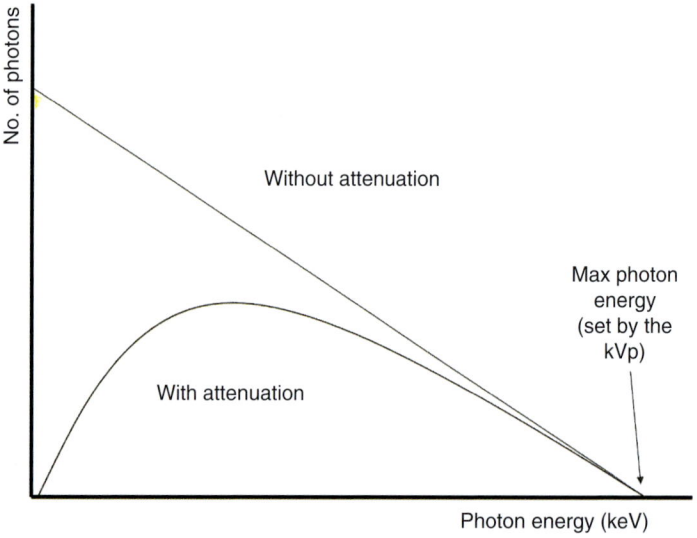

Figure 2.7 A plot of the number of photons versus their energy, in kiloelectron volts (keV). The straight line shows the number produced in the target, that is, without attenuation and the curved line shows the number of photons in the beam on exiting the target and X-ray tube, that is, with attenuation. Note that characteristic radiation is not shown as those peaks are dependent on the target material and kVp selected.

- Characteristic interactions: If a high-velocity electron strikes and ejects an inner shell electron of the target atom, an outer shell electron in a higher-energy state will fill the inner shell vacancy, which is at a lower energy state. In doing so, EM radiation is emitted that is characteristic of the atom, and the shells of the ejected and outer shell electrons.

Target material: The target of an X-ray tube is the surface of the anode that is struck by the high-velocity electrons to make X-ray photons. Most mammography manufacturers choose to use molybdenum, rhodium, or tungsten as the target material. Further, most mammography units have the ability for more than one target material to be selected. The target material is chosen for several main properties. They are

- A high atomic number. The higher the number the greater the amount of bremsstrahlung radiation that is produced, that is, a greater conversion efficiency
- A high melting point
- High thermal capacity, that is, the ability to store heat
- Thermal conductivity, that is, the ability to transfer heat
- Appropriate K/L shell energies for the production of characteristic X-rays

Molybdenum was the most common material prior to the development and introduction of tomosynthesis in mammography, which is discussed in detail in Chapter 4. Table 2.3 shows some of the main characteristics of these target materials.

Some properties of mammography X-ray tube targets are as follows:

- Tungsten has a higher melting point and a higher atomic number, giving significantly more efficient X-ray production than molybdenum and rhodium.

Table 2.3 Typical Mammography X-Ray Tube Target Specifications.

Target Material	Molybdenum	Rhodium	Tungsten
Chemical symbol/ atomic number	Mo/42	Rh/45	W/74
Melting point	2,623°C	1964°C	3,422°C
Characteristic energies	K shell energies: 17.5–19.5 keV	K shell energies: 20.5–22.5 keV	L shell energies: approx. 12 keV
Relative X-ray output (compared to Mo)	1	1.15	3

- Molybdenum has K shell characteristic radiation at X-ray energies appropriate for small to medium-sized/ density breasts.
- Rhodium has K shell characteristic radiation at X-ray energies appropriate for medium to large size/density breasts. It also has slightly more efficient X-ray production than molybdenum.

The characteristic X-ray energies are determined by the energy difference between the orbital electron shells' energies and are unique for every material. The X-ray energies of molybdenum and rhodium are in a range that is desirable for many mammographic examinations, though some manufacturers are moving away from molybdenum and rhodium. The effects of characteristic radiation are discussed later in this chapter.

Anode angle: All modern X-ray tubes have angled or beveled anodes. The main purpose of this is to reduce the amount of attenuation of the X-ray photons prior to exiting the target itself. If the anode was not beveled and at 90° to the direction of the electron beam, the X-ray photons would travel a long distance through the anode and target material prior to exiting the X-ray tube.

In all X-ray production, the beam that exits the X-ray tube is divergent from the target. In general X-ray imaging, the central ray of the divergent X-ray beam is usually positioned perpendicular to the center of the image plate or detector. However, in mammography, this approach is not used. The X-ray tube and anode are angled relative to the image plate/detector so that one edge of the divergent is perpendicular to the edge of the image plate on the plate's chest wall side, as shown in Figures 2.2 and 2.4. Having a perpendicular or vertical beam at the edge of the image plate minimizes missed breast tissue near the chest wall that would occur if the beam was divergent from the center of the image plate.

With any angled or beveled anode, there are associated effects with the X-ray beam. They are the anode heel effect and variable focal spot size across the X-ray beam, best described using the line focus principle.

- Anode heel effect: X-ray photons are produced at depth in the target. Many high-velocity electrons will travel past surface atoms prior to interacting with an atom to produce bremsstrahlung or characteristic X-ray photons. As shown in Figure 2.5a and b, the distance the photon has to travel to exit the target is greatest on the anode end of the target and least on the cathode end. Further a photon travels through any material, in this case, the target material; the greater the probability of the photon interacting with atoms of that material and hence greater attenuation will occur. As such, the intensity of the X-ray beam decreases from its maximal value on the cathode side of the field to the anode side of the field. In Figure 2.5a and b, two orientations of the X-ray tube are seen. One orientation is the cathode, which is toward the chest wall, and the other is the anode, which is toward the chest wall. The advantage of having the cathode of the X-ray tube toward the chest wall is that the greatest intensity in the X-ray beam will travel through the thickest part of the breast at the chest wall.

■ Variable focal spot size (from the line focus principle) across the X-ray field: The line focus principle describes the relationship between the filament size, the angle of the target, and the size of the effective focal spot. The effective focal spot size is that dimension of the actual focal spot that can be "seen" from the image plate and it varies in size across the X-ray field. The length of the dimension projected on the image plate, hence the effective focal spot, is smallest on the cathode side of the X-ray field. A smaller effective focal spot size will increase the spatial resolution of the ability to see detail in the image. In Figure 2.5c and d, two orientations of the X-ray tube are seen. One orientation is so the cathode, which is toward the chest wall, and the other is the anode, which is toward the chest wall. The advantage of having the anode of the X-ray tube toward the chest wall is the smallest effective focal spot size, and hence the greatest detail, which will be seen in the thickest part of the breast at the chest wall.

Manufacturers of mammography units will choose the anode/cathode orientation that they think best suits their unit. However, the most common orientation is to have the cathode toward the chest wall to maximize the beam's intensity near the chest wall.

The anode angle determines the relationship between the cathode filament and the actual focal spot on the target to create the projected or effective focal spot, which is a factor in determining the spatial resolution of the image.

■ A large anode angle produces a larger projected focal spot size and poor spatial resolution and image detail, however, the X-ray field size coverage can be larger.

- A smaller anode angle results in a smaller projected focal spot size and better spatial resolution and image detail; however, the X-ray field size coverage will be smaller.
- The following are some details regarding anode angles:
    - In general X-ray imaging, the X-ray tubes typically have a range of anode angles of 6–13°.
    - In mammography, the X-ray tubes typically have a range of anode angles of 20–22°. These angles are usually the sum of two angles (see Figures 2.2 and 2.4) being
        - the angle of the anode within the tube and the tilt of the X-ray tube is typically 4–6°.
        - one notable exception by one manufacturer, which has a unique design, has an anode with zero degrees anode angle and a 22° tube tilt.
    - Some manufacturers provide a different anode angle for the large and small focal spots. A bi-angle tube with an anode with two different angles is used for the large and small focal spots. The angle for the small focal spot is typically 9–10° less than for the large focal spot. The small anode angle is always used with the small focal spot, and the larger anode angle is used with the large focal spot.
- Added to the use of bi-angled anode is that some manufacturers will have anode tracks also made from different materials, for example, molybdenum, rhodium, or tungsten.

X-ray tube window: An exit port or window in the X-ray tube is needed that is strong enough to contain the vacuum in the X-ray tube while offering as little attenuation as possible to the low-energy X-ray photons needed for mammography. The window or exit port material used in modern mammography is beryllium with the atomic symbol of Be. Beryllium has an atomic number of only 4 and a density of 1.8, which are both the lowest for any metal. The thickness of the beryllium in the window is typically 0.8–1.0 mm.

X-ray filters: Filters, made of various metals or in some cases other solid materials, are placed in the path of the X-ray beam as the beam exits the X-ray tube window. In general X-ray imaging, the material is typically aluminum, and its purpose is to remove the low-energy photons from the beam prior to the photons reaching the patient. These low-energy photons have little to no possibility of contributing to the image but would only contribute to patient dose, particularly skin dose. Figure 2.7 shows the attenuated beam, the curved line in the plot, after the X-ray beam has exited the tube and passed through the anode/target and filter material. The total filtration in any diagnostic X-ray system, including mammography, must be greater than or equal to 0.5 mm aluminum equivalent to satisfy most countries' regulations. This does not mean that aluminum must be used as the filter; however, whatever material is used, its attenuation of the X-ray beam must be at least as much as would be achieved using 0.5 mm of aluminum.

All X-ray beams produced in an X-ray tube are polychromatic, that is, there is a broad range of photon energies in the beam. The curved line plot in Figure 2.7 shows the attenuated beam as it exits the X-ray tube. It has a range of photon energies from the maximum photon energy, set by the kVp across the X-ray tube, to low photon energies. In mammography, filtration has a second and just as important purpose as the removal of low-energy photons from the beam. The second purpose is to "shape" the beam. The "shaping" of the beam or spectrum means to selectively remove certain photon energies from the beam so the beam's range of photon energies is reduced or concentrated, and the mean or average energy of the beam's spectrum can be altered depending on the filter material.

The means of attenuating or reducing selectively a range of photon energies in the beam is done by selecting the appropriate filter material. All materials have inner shell electrons, and most will have other shells of electrons. These shells are labeled the K-shell for the innermost and L-shell, M-shell, etc. for outer shells depending on the material. The electrons in the atom's shells are bound to the nucleus of the atom and the binding energy of the electron is specific to that material. Given a range of photon energies passing through matter, the photons with higher energy will be less attenuated than those with lower energies. This is shown in Figure 2.8b as a decrease in attenuation as photon energy increases, in kilo-electron volts (keV). As X-ray photons pass through the material, they must have an energy greater than the binding energy to break the shell's electron bond with the nucleus. X-ray photons with energies below the binding energy will be attenuated by coherent or Compton attenuation processes. However, when the photon energies match or just exceed the shell electron's binding energy, attenuation increases as these photons can break that bond and eject that shell electron from the atom. This is shown in Figure 2.8b as a sharp increase in attenuation as photon energy increases and is the photoelectric effect. For K-shell electrons, this is known as the K-edge of the material.

Figure 2.8a shows the X-ray spectrum from a molybdenum target, with both the bremsstrahlung and characteristic photons, as it exits the X-ray tube prior to passing through the filter. The attenuation curve of the filter material, also molybdenum, is shown in Figure 2.8b and the resultant attenuated/filtered from the molybdenum/molybdenum spectrum is shown in Figure 2.8c. This spectrum is both attenuated at lower and higher photon energies and, as a result, has a narrower range of photon energies in the desired energy range needed for that examination.

Matching of the target material and the filter material is important. The K-edge of the filter should not be lower than the characteristic spectral peaks, or these photons will be attenuated and removed from the beam.

Commonly used filter materials are molybdenum, rhodium, silver, and aluminum and some manufacturers use copper. Table 2.4 provides the main specifications of these filter materials. Table 2.5 shows a combination of anode material and filter material that can be used and materials that are commonly used in mammography units.

In Figure 2.9, the attenuation curves of molybdenum (dark line) and rhodium (lighter line) with their two different K-edges of 20.0 and 23.2 keV are compared. Using a target/filter

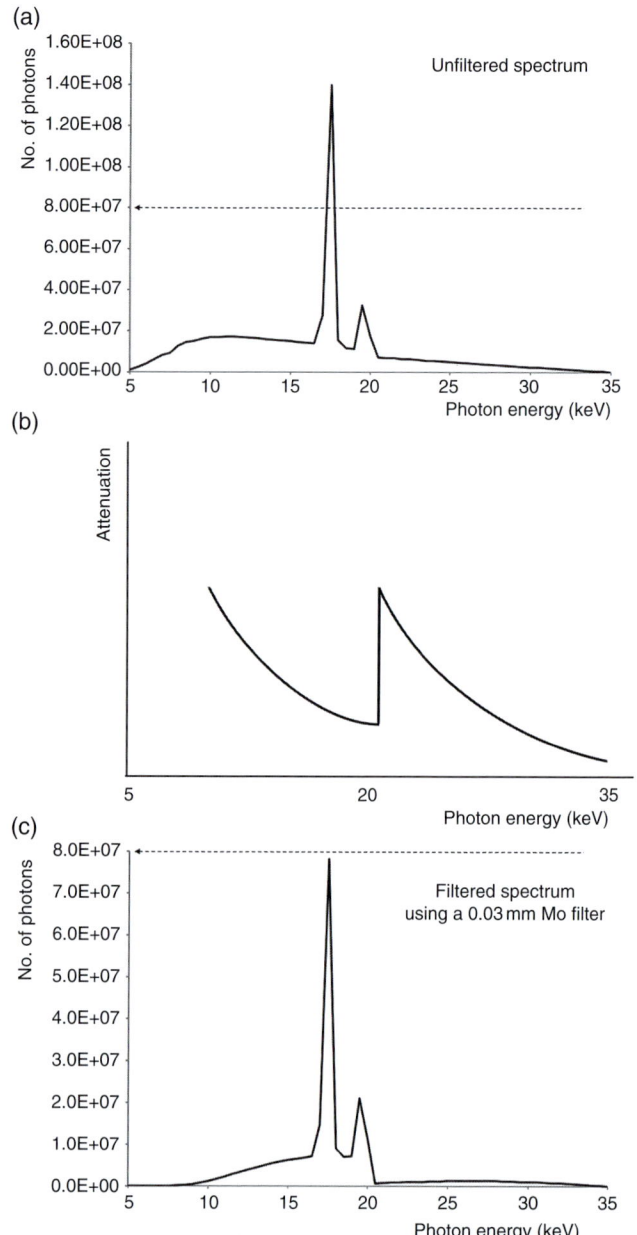

Figure 2.8 (a) X-ray spectrum from a molybdenum target, unfiltered as it exits the tube, showing both the bremsstrahlung photon curve and characteristic photon peaks. (b) Attenuation plot of a molybdenum filter showing a K-edge at 20.0 keV. (c) Resultant X-ray spectrum after the beam passes through 0.03 mm thickness of a molybdenum filter. Dashed horizontal lines at 80 million photons compare the scale of the Y-axis between (a) and (c). Spectrum plots were created using the Boone Normalized Glandular Dose (DgN) and spectrum calculator. *Source:* Adapted from Boone, Fewell et al. (1997) and Boone (2002).

Table 2.4 Typical Mammography X-ray Filter Materials and Specifications.

Filter Material	Aluminum	Copper	Molybdenum	Rhodium	Silver
Chemical symbol/atomic number	Al/13	Cu/29	Mo/42	Rh/45	Ag/47
K-edge	1.5 keV	9.0 keV	20.0 keV	23.2 keV	25.5 keV
Typical filter thicknesses	0.7 mm	0.3 mm	0.025–0.03 mm	0.025–0.05 mm	0.03–0.05 mm

Table 2.5 Typical Mammography Target/Filter Combinations.

Target Materials		Molybdenum	Rhodium	Tungsten
Acceptable filter materials with the target	Molybdenum	✓		
	Rhodium	✓	✓	✓
	Silver	✓	✓	✓
	Aluminum	✓	✓	✓
Commonly used filter materials with the target	Molybdenum	✓		
	Rhodium	✓	✓	✓
	Silver		✓	✓
	Aluminum			✓

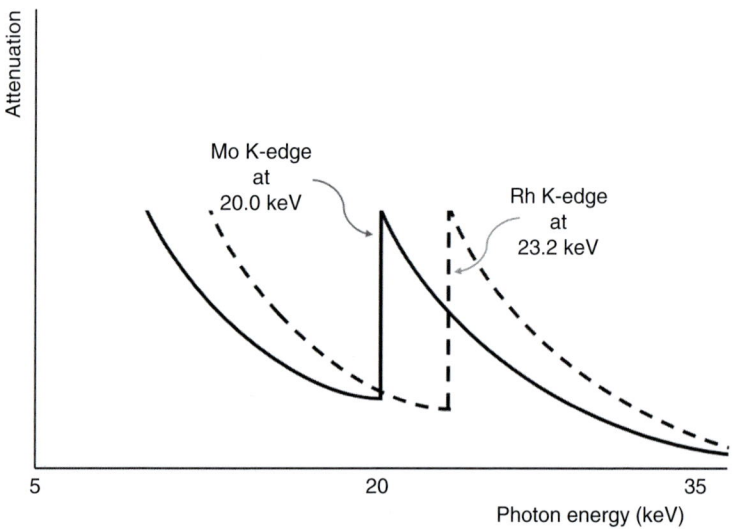

Figure 2.9 Attenuation curves comparison from a molybdenum filter (solid line) and a rhodium filter (dashed line) showing their K-edges of 20.0 and 23.2 keV, respectively.

combination of molybdenum/rhodium will, without increasing the X-ray tube voltage, create a beam with a higher average energy than using a target/filter combination of molybdenum/ molybdenum.

In general X-ray imaging, the prime method of increasing the X-ray beam's average photon energy is to increase the kVp. Increasing kVp increases both the beam's average energy and the number of photons produced. Figure 2.10 shows an example of increasing the beam's average energy by using a different filter to increase the average energy of the X-ray beam compared to the resultant beam in Figure 2.8c. Figure 2.10a is the spectral plot from a molybdenum target that was shown in Figure 2.8a. Figure 2.10b shows the attenuation curves, also shown in Figure 2.9, of both molybdenum and rhodium filters. When placing a rhodium filter, with a K-edge of 23.2 keV, in the beam compared to the molybdenum filter, with a K-edge of 20.0 keV, the resultant plot from molybdenum target and rhodium filter is shown in Figure 2.10c. This shows an increase in the number of photons above 20.0 keV, compared to Figure 2.8c.

Increasing kVp also increases the number of photons produced. The so-called 15% kVp rule states that the number of photons is approximately doubled when the kVp is increased by 15%. In mammography, changing the anode and filter selections is the main means of changing the average energy of the X-ray beam.

In Figure 2.11, a plot that would result from a tungsten target and a silver filter, with the vertical line of the K-edge at 25.5 keV is seen. Note that in the plot, no characteristic energies are seen. Tungsten's K shell energies are above the kVp set for mammography, whereas the L shell energies are typically removed by the filter material and the anode itself as the photons exit the anode.

Increasing the kVp, using the same target/filter combination, does slightly increase the beam's average energy; however, the main result is an increase in the number of X-ray photons

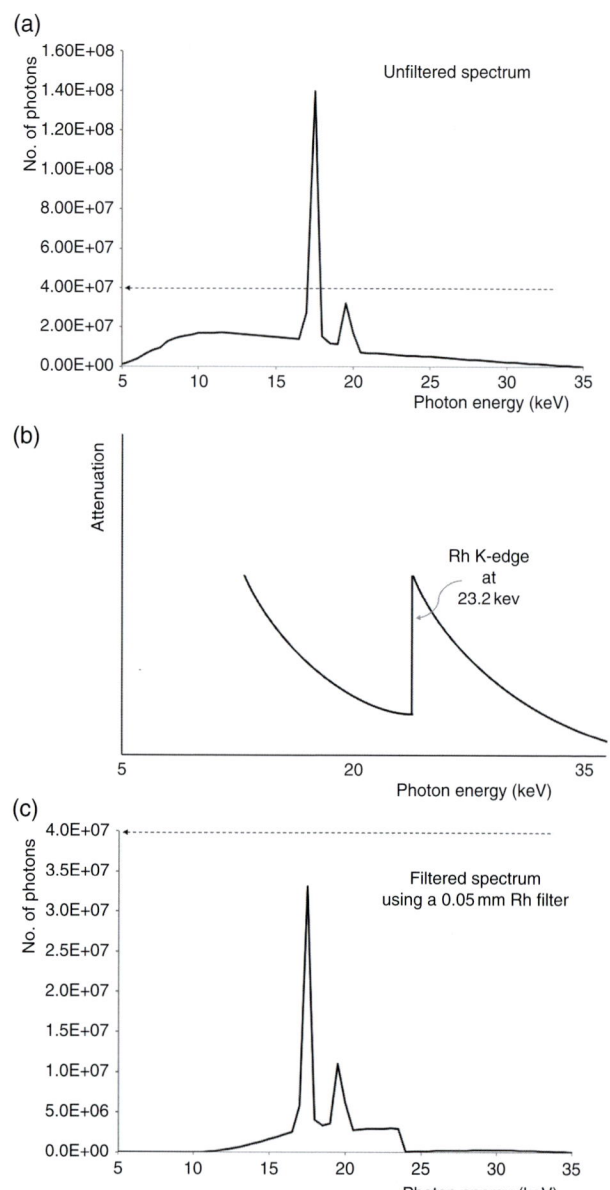

Figure 2.10 (a) X-ray spectrum from a molybdenum target, unfiltered as it exits the tube, showing both the bremsstrahlung photon curve and characteristic photon peaks. (b) Attenuation plot of a rhodium filter showing a K-edge at 23.2 keV. (c) Resultant X-ray spectrum after the beam passes through 0.05 mm thickness of a rhodium filter. Dashed horizontal line at 40 million photons compares the scale of the Y-axis between (a) and (c). Note: the increase of the number of photons between 20.0 and 23.2 keV compared to the Mo/Mo plot in Figure 2.8c. Spectrum plots were created using the Boone Normalized Glandular Dose (DgN) and spectrum calculator.
Source: Adapted from Boone, Fewell et al. (1997) and Boone (2002).

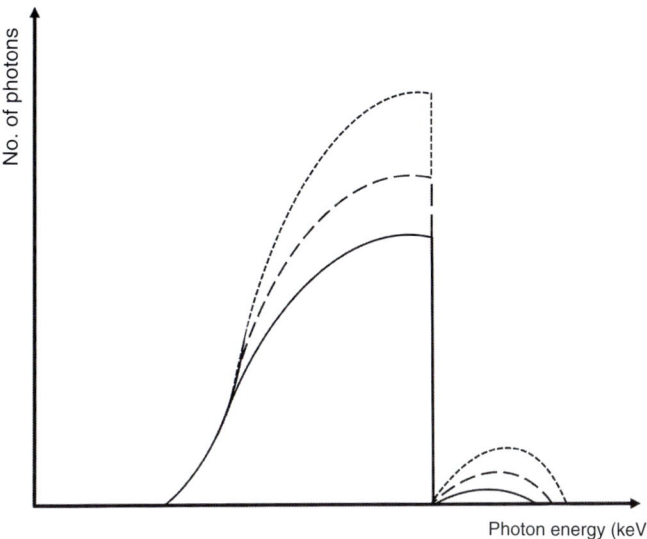

Figure 2.11 X-ray spectrum from a tungsten target, using a silver filter (K-edge = 25.5 keV) at three kVp settings. The solid line is the lowest kVp setting; the dashed line is the middle kVp setting; and the dotted line is at the highest kVp setting.

produced. The solid line in Figure 2.11 shows the beam with the lowest kVp setting, the dashed line is the middle kVp setting, and the dotted line is the beam with the largest kVp setting. The filter attenuates the photon above its K-edge, so there is only a small increase in higher-energy photons, however, the main effect of increasing kVp is shown with an increase in the number of photons.

Beam limitation (collimation): In the early days of mammography, the X-ray beam was limited to the breast being imaged using either movable blades or D-shaped diaphragms. The disadvantage of this type of collimation is that much of the image was clear, providing a bright background and reducing the displayed or observed image contrast. Modern mammography units collimate the X-ray beam to the size of the flat panel detector. Unattenuated X-rays reaching the image plate result in high image pixel values that are displayed as black in the image. Having a black background around the breast anatomy improves overall displayed image contrast and it becomes easier for clinicians to view and visualize subtle features of the image. Other factors are:

- the patient dose remains the same.
- there is no increase in scattered radiation since the whole breast is irradiated both when using D-shaped diaphragms and collimating to the entire flat panel detector.

Accurate collimation is most critical at the chest wall side of the X-ray beam. This is a unique requirement for mammography which is discussed earlier.

Geometry: Figures 2.1 and 2.2 show the arrangement of the X-ray tube, collimator, compression paddle, breast support, grid, and image receptor. Patient positioning and imaging geometry are two important aspects of setting up a mammography examination. Imaging geometry refers to the spatial relationship of the X-ray source, patient, and the image receptor. There are several unique aspects of mammography imaging geometry as compared with general radiography:

The source to image distance (SID): In mammography, this is a short distance than is typically used in general X-ray imaging, that of 100 cm (40 in.) for most examinations and 180 cm (70 in.) for several other examinations. Some mammography details are:-

Source–image distance (SID):

- 65–70 cm is typical.
- SID effects:
  - X-ray photon intensity: If the SID was 100 cm, the inverse square law relationship with distance, the SID, means lower radiation intensity would reach the breast for a given output of the X-ray tube. To

compensate for that, either a high mA (noting the maximum mA settings for the smaller mammography focal spot sizes) or a longer exposure time would be needed, risking motion blur in the image.

■ Geometric unsharpness (penumbra): A small focal spot size in mammography is needed with short SIDs to reduce object geometric unsharpness in the image (which appears as blurred edges in the image). With a SID of 100 cm, a larger focal spot size can be tolerated as magnification of an object in the image increases geometric unsharpness.

■ Skin dose: Shorter SID results in a higher skin dose for a given dose to the image receptor.

Source–object distance (SOD):

■ Is equal to breast tissue thickness plus breast support – image plate distance (several millimeters).

■ Is greater for structures that are closer to the X-ray tube than for structures that are closer to the image plate.

Image magnification:

■ Image magnification (M) = SID/SOD or SID/(SID − OID) (object to image distance).

■ Magnification increases as the distance between the object and the image plate increases.

■ Magnification of objects in the image occurs in all X-ray imaging as there is a divergent X-ray beam and the object never is directly in contact with the image receptor (there will always be some distance thickness of the image receptor cover).

■ In mammography, 5–10% magnification (M = 1.05–1.10) is the typical standard for the so-called non-magnification imaging.

■ In breast and all X-ray imaging, structures closer to the X-ray tube will have higher image magnification than structures closer to the image plate.

In mammography, geometric magnification, as opposed to image magnification, is sometimes used to deliberately enlarge the image of structures in the breast. This is usually referred to as magnification mammography where the breast is positioned on a magnification platform at a large OID.

■ Manufacturers will provide platforms to support the breast typically at several magnification factors of 1.5 and 1.8 and sometimes 2.0.

    ■ For a magnification factor of 1.5 at a SID of 65 cm, the magnification platform will be approximately 21.7 cm from the image plate.

    ■ For a magnification factor of 1.8 at a SID of 65 cm, the magnification platform will be approximately 28.9 cm from the image plate.

■ If the magnification platform is labeled M = 1.5, most of the breast is imaged at a magnification greater than 1.5 because of the thickness of the breast.

■ When performing a magnification view, a small focal spot must be used to decrease geometric unsharpness (formerly known as penumbra).

■ The small focal spot requires a reduction in tube current (see earlier).

■ A low mA means a longer exposure time. Exposure times can be as long as several seconds or even more for magnification mammography on some patients.

■ With increasing magnification, an increasing geometric unsharpness is observed in the image. Excessive magnification will make the image larger but not sharper.

■ A specific spot compression paddle is used to compress a small portion of the breast, not the whole breast.

■ Collimation is restricted and reduced to the size of the spot compression paddle.

Half-field geometry is a unique but important feature of all modern mammography imaging systems (see Figure 2.2). In half-field geometry:

- The focal spot is directly above the chest wall edge of the breast support rather than being placed over the center of the anatomy to be imaged as it is typically for general radiography.
- The central ray of the X-ray beam is at right angles to the chest edge of the image plate and parallel to the chest wall of the patient.
- Half-field imaging is accomplished by angling the tube away from the patient.

In the diverging beam approach used in general X-ray imaging, the X-ray tube focus/central ray is typically centered in the middle of the image plate; in mammography, this approach would exclude some breast tissue from being imaged. Figure 2.12 shows an example of when the X-ray tube focus/central ray is centered in the middle of the image plate and the excluded breast tissue. As it is important to include all of the breast tissue in the mammogram, this divergence beam approach with the central ray over the middle of the image plate would be undesirable. Therefore, effective mammography requires half-field geometry.

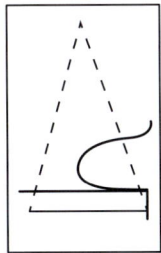

Figure 2.12 A diverging beam approach showing missed anatomy at the chest wall when the X-ray tube focus/central ray is centered in the middle of the image plate.

Compression: Compression of the breast is a further example of a major difference in imaging methods compared to general X-ray imaging. In general X-ray imaging, there are only a few instances of examinations, and a decrease in frequency all the time, where compression is used. Yet in mammography, compression is used in all examinations.

These benefits of compression in mammography include:

- Decreased breast thickness results in the following:
    - Lower radiation dose
    - Shorter exposure time
    - Less scattered radiation, which results in higher image contrast
- More uniform breast tissue thickness. As a result, density differences in the image from the edge of the breast to the center are reduced by improving overall image quality.
- Improved tissue structural visualization from tissue spreading.
- Reduced penumbra/increased image sharpness from decreased OID and resulting magnification.
- Decreased potential for motion due to the compression aiding in immobilization.

Some important technical capabilities for breast compression, most are as set out by the US Food and Drug Administration (FDA) in the Mammography Quality Standards Act (MQSA) and followed and accepted by most countries, that a mammography imaging system should have are:

- Initial power-driven compression activated by hands-free controls operable from both sides of the patient.
- Manual adjustment of compression from both sides of the patient.
- A compression force of at least 111 N (25 pounds).
- The maximum compression force for the initial power drive is between 111 and 200 N (25–45 pounds).

- Smooth, uniform application of compression force.
- Compression paddle should be flat and parallel to the breast support (within 1 cm for all corners) to satisfy MQSA requirements.
- Chest wall edge of paddle should be straight and parallel to the breast support.
- There should be a wall on the paddle at the patient side to keep unwanted tissue and skin out of the image.
- The wall should be parallel to the chest wall (perpendicular to the breast support) and have a smooth, rounded corner for patient comfort.
- The compression paddle must not be visible in the image at the chest wall.
- The compression paddle must not extend more than 1% of the SID beyond the chest wall edge of the image plate.
- There must be a properly sized compression paddle for each image plate size.
- Compression should be maintained until released at the end of the X-ray exposure.
- There must be a manual release of compression in case of a power failure.
- Spot compression paddles should be available for both standard and magnification imaging.
- Automatic decompression and raising of the paddle on termination of the exposure.

Breast support: The breast support, which is located between the Bucky grid and the breast, supports the breast and is the lower component of the compression mechanism to allow the compression force. Desirable features of breast supports are as follows:

- Low attenuation of the transmitted X-ray beam
- Sturdy: The support must not bow under the compression force or encroach on the motion of the grid.

- Carbon fiber is preferred: When manufactured improperly, however, the carbon fiber pattern can be visible in the image.
- Smooth edges and a compact design.

Chapter 3 will continue reviewing the physical principles in mammography, however, with a focus on mammographic image formation.

Bibliography

Böke, A. (2024). "Calculation of x-ray attenuation coefficients for normal and cancerous breast tissues." *Nuclear Engineering and Technology* 56(1): 241–246.

Boone, J. M. (2002). "Normalized glandular dose (DgN) coefficients for arbitrary x-ray spectra in mammography: computer-fit values of Monte Carlo derived data." *Medical Physics* 29(5): 869–875.

Boone, J. M., Fewell, T. R. and Jennings, R. J. (1997). "Molybdenum, rhodium, and tungsten anode spectral models using interpolating polynomials with application to mammography." *Medical Physics* 24(12): 1863–1874.

Bushong, S. C. (2021). *Radiologic Science for Technologists.* Mosby.

Fico, N., Di Grezia, G., Cuccurullo, V., Salvia, A. A. H., Iacomino, A., Sciarra, A. and Gatta, G. (2023). "Breast imaging physics in mammography (Part I)." *Diagnostics (Basel)* 13(20).

Fico, N., Grezia, G. D., Cuccurullo, V., Salvia, A. A. H., Iacomino, A., Sciarra, A., La Forgia, D. and Gatta, G. (2023). "Breast imaging physics in mammography (Part II)." *Diagnostics* 13(23): 3582.

Fredenberg, E., Willsher, P., Moa, E., Dance, D. R., Young, K. C. and Wallis, M. G. (2018). "Measurement of breast-tissue x-ray attenuation by spectral imaging: fresh and fixed normal and malignant tissue." *Physics in Medicine & Biology* 63(23): 235003.

Haus, A. G., Metz, C. E., Chiles, J. T. and Rossmann, K. (1976). "The effect of x-ray spectra from molybdenum and tungsten target tubes on image quality in mammography." *Radiology* 118(3): 705–709.

Kalaf, J. M. (2014). "Mammography: a history of success and scientific enthusiasm." *Radiologia Brasileira* 47(4): Vii-viii.

Soares, L. D. H., Gobo, M. S. S. and Poletti, M. E. (2020). "Measurement of the linear attenuation coefficient of breast tissues using polienergetic x-ray for energies from 12 to 50 keV and a silicon dispersive detector." *Radiation Physics and Chemistry* 167: 108226.

Tomal, A., Mazarro, I., Kakuno, E. M. and Poletti, M. E. (2010). "Experimental determination of linear attenuation coefficient of normal, benign and malignant breast tissues." *Radiation Measurements* 45(9): 1055–1059.

3 Mammography Image Formation

Chapter at a Glance

Digital Mammography: Physics and Instrumentation, Second Edition.
Rob Davidson.
© 2026 John Wiley & Sons Ltd. Published 2026 by John Wiley & Sons Ltd.

Introduction

Chapter 2 provided an overview of mammography instrumentation and looked at X-ray production. This chapter continues the X-ray photons' journey of interactions in the breast tissue, the control of when they scatter, to the important part of mammography, image recording and display.

The focus of these two chapters is on planar imaging, commonly called 2D mammography. However, many of these aspects are also relevant to advanced techniques including digital breast tomosynthesis (DBT), the so-called 3D mammography. The principles of DBT and other advanced techniques are discussed in Chapter 4.

Interaction of X-rays with Breast Tissue

As X-ray photons pass through any matter, one of three events happens. The events are:

- Transmission: The X-ray photons do not interact with any of the atoms in the matter, in this case, breast tissue. These photons pass through the matter and produce the final image when interacting with the image plate/flat panel detector.
- Scatter: The X-ray photons interact with atoms in the breast tissue, change direction, and lose energy. These

photons may travel without any further interactions within the breast tissue and exit the breast. If traveling in the forward direction, they may be detected by the flat panel detector and contribute to the value of the pixel. Alternatively, multiple scattering events may occur, and the photon gives up its entire energy after several interactions, which then becomes absorption.

■ Absorption: The X-ray photons give up their entire energy, either in a single or multiple events, in the breast tissue.

The last two processes, scatter and absorption collectively, are attenuation of the X-ray beam. These two processes contribute to deciding the radiation dose for the patient. They are necessary as differing tissue types, densities, and thicknesses produce the differential attenuation that is needed to create image contrast and allow the viewer to visualize different objects or anatomical regions in the image. However, these events are the causes of the radiation dose to the patient.

Scattered X-ray photons, if they reach the flat panel detector and are recorded, do not provide any information as to the differential attenuation from within the breast. An increase in photon numbers from scatter that reaches a flat panel detector increases overall pixel values, which when viewed as an image reduces image contrast. As such, scatter reaching the flat panel detector degrades image quality.

Attenuation of X-rays

The attenuation of an X-ray beam refers to the removal of photons from the beam as it passes through an object. During routine mammography, approximately 95% of the incident photons are attenuated by the breast. In mammography, attenuation of X-ray photons occurs by two mechanisms, photoelectric absorption and Compton scatter.

With **photoelectric absorption**, the incoming X-ray photon is absorbed by an atom and delivers all of its energy to an inner electron, ejecting it from the atom.

■ The X-ray photon gives up its energy to the atom and electrons, and the photon is removed completely from the beam.

■ Photoelectric interactions are beneficial to X-ray imaging because they are the most important source of image contrast.

■ The ejected electron carries away most of the energy of the incident X-ray photon and is the primary agent for depositing energy for the patient, which is the patient radiation dose.

■ The vacancy caused by the removal of the inner electron is filled by an outer electron causing a photon of radiation to be emitted. This new photon is characteristic of that atom. This is one source of scatter radiation.

■ The probability of photoelectric interaction increases with atomic number and decreases with energy, according to the following relationship:

$$\text{Probability of photoelectric interaction} \propto Z^3/E^3$$

where Z is the atomic number of the absorber; E is the photon energy.

■ Photoelectric interactions are dominant at low X-ray energies.

■ Mammographic imaging technology and techniques (target, filter, and tube voltage (peak kilovolt (kVp))) are chosen to provide a low-energy X-ray beam to maximize photoelectric attenuation.

In **Compton scatter**, the incoming photon interacts with an atom and shares its energy with an outer-shell electron.

■ The electron is ejected from the atom.
■ The photon persists but with diminished energy, and its direction is changed. This is another source of scatter radiation.
■ The scattered photon carries no information about the imaged breast and, if absorbed by the image receptor, it will decrease the image contrast.
■ Compton interactions
  ■ probability depends on the electron density (and therefore the tissue).
  ■ are relatively independent of energy
  ■ dominate at higher energies.

A comparison of photoelectric and Compton interactions at differing photon energies is shown in Figure 3.1.

Overall X-ray attenuation depends on the following factors:

■ X-ray beam's effective or average energy that depends on:
  ■ kVp
  ■ Voltage waveform (ripple factor)
  ■ Anode material
  ■ Filter material and thickness
■ Patient factors:
  ■ Breast thickness, which depends (within limits) on breast compression
  ■ Breast tissue density and composition
■ Other factors:
  ■ The compression paddle removes photons from the beam before breast exposure.
  ■ The breast support.

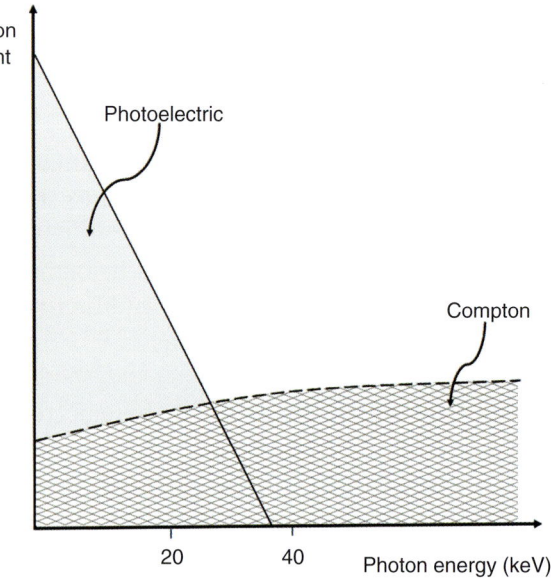

Figure 3.1 Photoelectric and Compton interactions at differing photon energies showing the predominance of photoelectric in the mammography range of X-ray photon energies.

■ The grid that removes approximately 50% of the primary photons from the beam after transmission through the breast.

Description of X-ray Attenuation

The effective energy of any diagnostic X-ray beam, including mammography, is conveniently measured and described by performing multiple measurements of the attenuation of the beam. The thickness of a material required to reduce the beam intensity to half is called the half-value layer (HVL) for that material. This is one of the main measures of the effective energy of the X-ray beam.

■ The HVL, at a given kVp setting, will vary depending on the target/filter combination selected. In mammography, given the same kVp setting, a target/filter combination of

   ■ tungsten (W)/silver (Ag) and tungsten (W)/ aluminum (Al) have the highest HVL's, and thus greater transmission through the breast tissue and the least radiation dose,

   ■ tungsten/rhodium (Rh) (W/Rh), and molybdenum/ rhodium (Mo/Rh) have lower HVLs, and

   ■ molybdenum/molybdenum (Mo/Mo) target/filter combination has the lowest HVL.

■ Typical HVL in mammography for a target/filter combination of Mo/Mo is approximately 0.33 mm of aluminum.

   ■ For soft tissue, the HVL is approximately 7 mm, which means that every 7 mm of tissue traversed by the beam reduces its intensity by one-half.

   ■ Example: A 4.2 cm breast is approximately 6 HVL (42 mm divided by 7 mm). Each HVL cuts the beam intensity in half, thus 6 HVLs transmit approximately 1.5% of the beam for the exit beam intensity.

   ■ This process is one definition of exponential attenuation and is illustrated for a 4.2-cm breast in Table 3.1.

This process is expressed mathematically as:

$$\text{Transmission} = \left(1/2\right)^{N}$$

where N is the number of HVLs traversed by the beam. In the example above:

$$\left(1/2\right)^{6} = 0.015 = 1.5\%$$

Table 3.1 The Number of X-ray Photons and Percentage of Transmission from an Initial One Million Photons at Various Thickness of Breast Tissue for a Target/Filter Combination of Molybdenum/Molybdenum (Mo/Mo).

Transmitted through:	# of Photons	Transmission (%)
Input: 1,000,000 X-ray photons		
0.7 cm of breast tissue	500,000	50.0
1.4 cm of breast tissue	250,000	25.0
2.1 cm of breast tissue	125,000	12.5
2.8 cm of breast tissue	63,000	6.3
3.5 cm of breast tissue	31,000	3.1
4.2 cm of breast tissue	15,000	1.5
Output	**15,000**	**1.5**

Differential Attenuation or Absorption/ Subject Contrast

The difference in radiation attenuation or absorption between tissues being imaged is often referred to as differential attenuation or absorption and it is also called subject contrast. This characteristic of tissues is important because of its significant contribution to image contrast, prior to the image undergoing post-processing in a computer. In mammography the:

- contrast of a tumor or calcification with surrounding normal breast tissue depends on the following factors:
    - The difference in atomic number (Z)
        - Z for all soft tissues is approximately 7
        - Z of calcium is 20
    - The difference in density
        - Density of fibroglandular tissues is approximately 1

- Density of adipose tissue is approximately 0.93
- Density of calcifications (calcium apatite) is approximately 3
- Gland-to-adipose contrast is mainly a result of density difference since the atomic numbers are similar
  - These attenuation differences are shown at different X-ray photon energies in Figure 1.1.
- thickness or diameter of the tumor or calcification
- tissue-to-calcium contrast as a result of the differences in density and Z
- type of surrounding tissue for mass lesions
  - Low contrast with glandular tissue (they are almost iso-dense)
  - Higher contrast when surrounded by adipose tissue
- image contrast is reduced by scattered radiation
- visibility of calcifications is also affected by the image noise

Controlling Scattered Radiation

Scattered or secondary radiation is a by-product of X-ray photons interacting with the breast tissue. Scattered radiation, when reaching the flat panel detector and contributing to the image, has the undesirable effect of reducing image contrast. In breast imaging, scattered radiation results from both photoelectric and Compton interactions. The intensity of scattered radiation primarily depends on the volume of tissue irradiated. The amount of scatter radiation is often measured as the scatter fraction (SF) which is the portion of scatter in the total amount of radiation that reaches the detector. For a breast thickness of 4 cm, the SF is 0.35–0.4, for 6 cm, it is approximately 0.45 and for 8 cm, thickness, 0.5–0.55. The primary beam is those X-ray photons that travel from the X-ray tube and through the breast to the image receptor, that are, are not scattered in the breast tissue. The primary beam carries the information that is desired to record in the image. Scattered radiation that is recorded on the image reduces image contrast and thereby reduces the diagnostic value of the exam. Reduction of scattered radiation is important and is accomplished in several ways.

Compression/Breast Thickness

The greater the path length (the distance a photon travels) through the object, the greater the probability that there will be an interaction between the photon and an atom in the object. With increasing breast thickness, as discussed earlier, there is an increasing amount of scatter radiation produced. One of the main objectives of compression in mammography is to reduce breast thickness, thus reducing the path length and the number of scattered photons that are created and then can potentially reach the flat panel detector and degrade image quality.

Collimation

In general radiography, an important method to reduce the amount of scatter radiation produced is to collimate the X-ray field tightly to the desired anatomy. As discussed previously, collimation is not used in standard mammographic image. As such, this is not a method of scatter reduction in standard 2D mammography.

However, in magnification mammography with a spot compression paddle, collimation is undertaken. With both tighter collimation and even further reduced breast thickness from the spot breast compression, less scatter is produced in magnification mammography, and this helps improve the resultant image quality.

Grids

The purpose of a grid is to reduce scattered radiation reaching the image receptor/flat panel detector. The grid is placed between the object being imaged and the flat panel detector. If the scatter is reduced or stopped from reaching the flat panel detector, image contrast and hence image quality is improved.

A grid is built by aligning a series of thin attenuating strips (usually lead or tantalum) such that the primary radiation can pass through while most of the scattered radiation is attenuated. In mammography, the attenuating strips are angled to align with the focal point of the X-ray target. The focal distance of the grid and source-to-image distance (SID) closely align, giving a minor variation in that the grid is placed on top of the flat panel detector. There are two main types of grids, the first type is with the linear attenuating strips that are parallel to each other, called a linear grid. Figure 3.2 shows a diagram of a linear grip with Figure 3.2a showing a front view and Figure 3.2b showing the

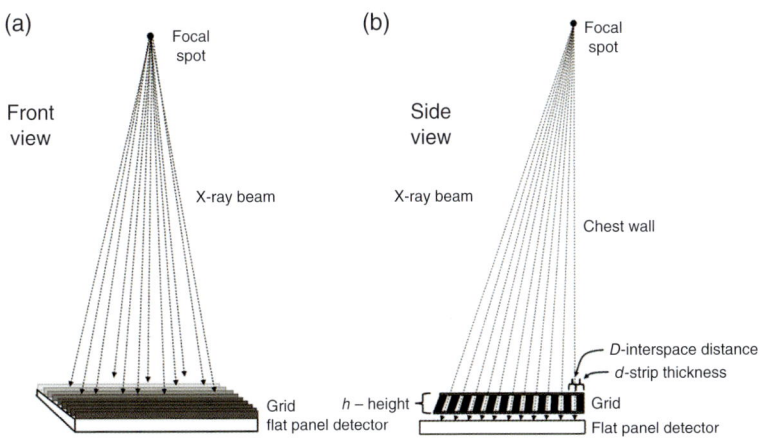

Figure 3.2 A diagrammatic representation of a linear grid. (a) The front view and the parallel attenuating strips and (b) the side view with the angled strips which have a focus at the X-ray target's focal point. Note that the diagrams are not to scale.

side-on view and angle of the attenuating strips. A mammography linear grid differs from a general radiography grid in that the vertical attenuating strips are at the edge of the grid, directly under the focal point of the target and on the chest wall edge of the grid, not in the center of the grid.

The spacer materials called the interspace material are placed between the attenuating strips and are required to hold the strips in place. Interspace material is made of a less attenuating material such as wood, plastic, or paper. Unfortunately, the material still attenuates the primary radiation to some level. One exception is the high transmission cellular (HTC) grid, used by one manufacturer. This grid has a rhombus-shaped structure with open space (air) between the septa. A diagrammatic representation of a HTC grid is shown in Figure 3.3. In general

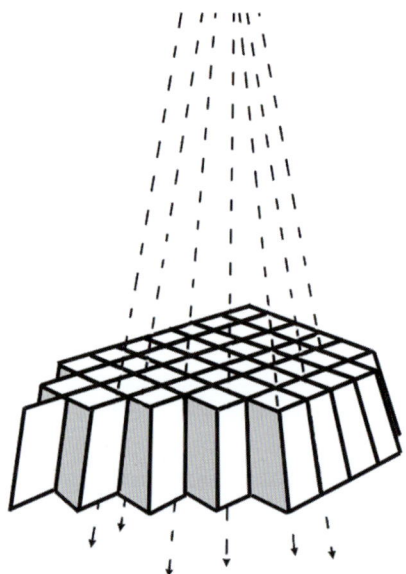

Figure 3.3 A diagrammatic representation of a High Transmission Cellular (HTC) grid with air, not a material, between the attenuating walls of the grid's septa. Note that the diagram is not to scale.

radiography, this is similar to a so-called crossed grid, which is essentially two linear grids, one on top of the other, but with the grid strips at a right angle to each other.

Both types of grids have features or characteristics, some of which are similar, and others differ. These are:

- The grid is positioned just underneath the breast support and above the image receptor.
- Scatter radiation is predominantly not traveling on the same angle/path as the primary radiation photons and strikes an inner wall of the attenuating strips (see Figure 3.4).

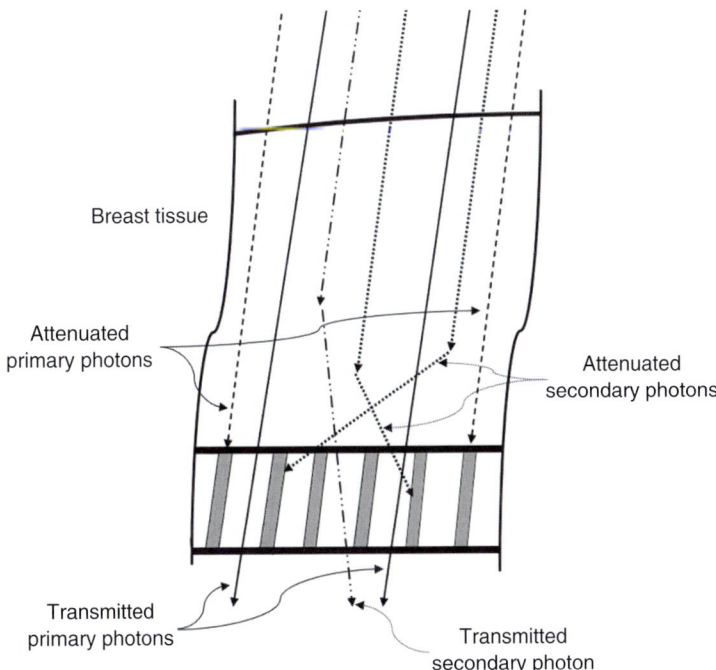

Figure 3.4 Primary and secondary (scattered) radiations either transmitting through the grid or being attenuated by the strips (Not to Scale).

- Primary radiation may strike the end of the attenuating strips rather than traveling through the interspace material. As such, the use of a grid reduces the amount of primary radiation reaching the flat panel detector (see Figure 3.4).
- A mammography grid typically attenuates:
    - About one-half of the primary radiation
    - Approximately 70–80% of the scattered radiation
- A grid improves image contrast but with a cost of increased dose due to the attenuation of the primary radiation and the need to compensate for this photon loss.
- A linear grid can be a moving grid using a Bucky mechanism.
    - The movement is designed to blur the grip strips, the image of which would cause artifacts in the mammographic image.
    - The movement is at right angles to the direction of the strips otherwise the movement would not blur the strips in the image.
    - As such, the grid has a focal range, a few centimeters plus/minus the SID of the unit.
    - A linear grid can be used in tomosynthesis.
- A HTC grid must be stationary, otherwise grid cut-off would increase. Grid cut-off occurs when the grid and the X-ray beam are incorrectly aligned, and the grid attenuates the primary beam more than when the grid and the X-ray beam are correctly aligned.
    - A HTC grid cannot be used in tomosynthesis. When tomosynthesis is selected, the HTC grid is removed from the X-ray beam
- A characteristic of a grid is the grid ratio (R), which is equal to the height of the strips divided by the distance between them (seen in Figure 3.2), written as:

$$\text{Ratio}\,(R) = h/d$$

where h is the height of the strips; d is the separation between the strips or the interspace distance.

- A typical grid ratio for mammography grids is 4:1 or 5:1. This ratio is considerably lower than regular general radiography grids which typically have R values between 8 and 12.
- High R grids will stop scatter radiation more effectively but typically also stop more primary radiation. Low R grids are used in mammography because of the low X-ray energies and less scatter being produced than, for example, compared to a human abdomen.
  Mammography grids must be thin, meaning that the h is small, to prevent excessive loss of primary radiation.
- Another characteristic of a grid is the grid frequency. This is the number of attenuating strips and interspace gaps divided by the distance. In mammography, grids are typically 60–80 lines/cm or 150–200 lines/in.

$$\text{Grid frequency} = (D + d)/\text{distance}$$

where D is the width of the strips; d is the separation between the strips or the interspace distance (shown in Figure 3.2).

  - The higher the frequency, the less visible the attenuating strips are on the image
- Carbon–fiber grid covers are preferred for their low attenuation.

The contrast improvement factor (CIF) is a measure of the effectiveness of a grid to remove scatter radiation compared to the scatter reaching the flat panel detector without a grid. It is measured as the ratio of image contrast with a grid to the ratio without a grid. For mammography, typical contrast improvement is 15–50%, depending on the grid and breast thickness (CIF = 1.15–1.50).

Because both scattered and primary radiations have been removed from the beam by the grid, the required X-ray exposure to produce the same number of X-ray photons reaching the flat panel detector increases. Exposure factors must be increased to maintain the same number of X-ray photons reaching the flat panel detector. The ratio of required exposure with the grid to the ratio without the grid is commonly referred to as the Bucky factor.

Typical Bucky factors for mammography grids are 2–3. This value means that using a grid increases the patient dose by a factor of 2–3 compared with no grid.

Air Gap

The air gap method can be used to reduce the amount of scatter reaching the flat panel detector. In the air gap method, the object-to-image distance (OID) is increased by creating a gap between the object being imaged and the flat panel detector. As such, the source-to-object distance (SOD) is reduced. Given the same point and angle of scatter in the object with no air gap and with an air gap, less scatter/secondary radiation will reach the flat panel detector using the air gap method, see Figure 3.5. A disadvantage of using an air gap in general radiography is increased magnification and penumbra (geometric unsharpness) and an increased chance of distortion of the object in the image. However, in mammography, magnification is sometimes used and has its advantages.

Magnification is used in mammography to improve the visualization of calcifications or other small, medium-to-high-contrast structures. In magnification mammography, the breast is moved approximately 30 cm (12 in.) away from the flat panel detector and closer to the X-ray source. The following are considerations for the use of this operating mode:

- Because the breast is moved closer to the X-ray source, the irradiated tissue receives a higher radiation dose when compared to standard mode imaging.

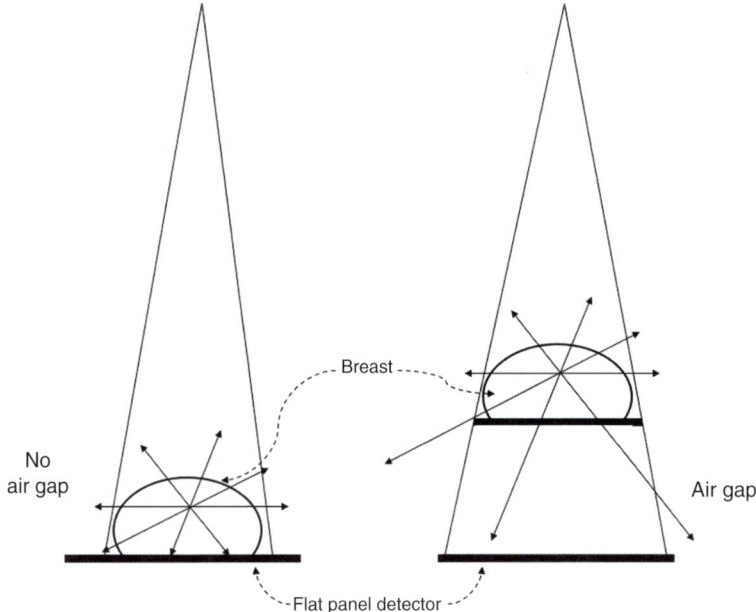

Figure 3.5 The air gap method increases the object-to-image distance creating a gap between the object being imaged and the flat panel detector. Given the same point and angle of scatter in the object in the no air gap and the air gap, less scatter/secondary radiation will reach the flat panel detector in the air gap method.

- Example: If the magnification factor is two, then the SOD is half of the original SOD, and the patient's dose increases, with the same exposure factors used originally. This is calculated using the 1/distance ^{2} rule and there is an increase in the patient's dose from the original dose to four times that dose.
- To compensate for this increase in the patient's radiation dose, the grid should be removed from the path of the X-ray beam. Removing the grid reduces the required exposure by the Bucky factor amount, typically two or three times. Without the grid and with reduced exposure factors, the patient's radiation dose is only slightly increased compared to non-magnification mode using a grid.

- The grid can be removed because the increase in OID creates an air gap, thereby reducing the contribution of scattered radiation to the image and the resultant reduction of image contrast.

Exposure Selection

All modern mammography units will enable the ability of the operator to select from a range of exposure modes. This range of exposure modes is greater than general radiography units. The names of these modes vary between manufacturers; however, they are similar in their approach to controlling the exposure parameters. The modes are:

- Manual: In manual mode, all exposure parameters of the kVp, milliampere-seconds (mAs), and target/filter combination are selected by the operator.
- Automatic timer: The kVp and target/filter combination are selected by the operator. The automatic exposure control (AEC) system will terminate the exposure when the desired amount of radiation is incident on the flat panel detector.
- Automatic filter: This mode can be used to identify the appropriate filter material for the selected target material to be used for that patient.
- Automatic kVp: This mode can be used to set the appropriate kVp for the set target/filter combination.

Automatic Exposure Control

Automatic exposure control (AEC) device when selected will terminate the exposure. An AEC is an ionization chamber; it operates by creating an electrical signal that is generated by an X-ray interaction, ionizations, in the device. Exposure termination occurs when the desired signal amount is received. In mammography, the AEC is located behind the flat panel detector. In general radiography, the AEC device is located in front of the flat panel detector. The requirement in mammography is low-energy X-ray photons due to low subject contrast in the breast tissue. If the AEC device was placed in front of the receptor, the device would create an artifact, undesired nonanatomical objects, in the image.

The AEC sensor will be moveable or will have several selectable locations for operator selection depending on the breast size and type. The AEC sensor must be highly sensitive since it receives only a small fraction of 1% of the X-ray radiation exiting the breast. Some important features that are desirable in an AEC are:

- Multiple sensors that give the AEC the capability of automatically finding the detector that is closest to the densest glandular tissue and then using the signal from the sensor (or combination of sensors) to terminate the exposure.
- Smart sensors that derive information about the energy of the X-ray beam and make corrections for the overall attenuation of the breast.
- An AEC circuit that can terminate the exposure quickly when it senses that the backup time will be reached. This feature prevents needless patient radiation dose.
- Accurate compensation for variations in breast thickness and kVp.
- Adjustable control that sets the AEC to receive a different amount of exposure.
- Accurate markings on the compression paddle that correspond to the AEC sensor locations.

Image Recording

History of Image Recording

When dedicated mammography units were introduced in the 1960s, conventional film-screen systems were used to record the image. These image systems suffered from blurred images due to the distance the light from the intensifying screen traveled to the film. Industrial film systems without intensifying screens were then used to improve spatial resolution/image detail and reduce image blur. The disadvantage of not using intensifying screens is a large increase in radiation dose.

In the early 1970s, a single intensifying screen with a single emulsion film in a vacuumized bag was introduced that reduced radiation dose and improved spatial resolution/image detail. Also, around this time, xeromammography was developed and introduced as an image recording medium. A xeromammography image is shown in Figure 3.6. Xeromammography was a paper image, not transparent film, and blue toner was used to coat the paper. Its process was based on Xerox photo-copying processes that were used at that time. A significant advantage was its inherent edge enhancement of objects in the image, enabling object edges to be easily visualized. However, spatial resolution/image detail was still poor.

In the mid-1970s, dedicated mammography film-screen combinations were introduced. These combinations produced sharper images and required approximately half of the radiation exposure of earlier film-screen combinations. Low attenuation cassettes, compared to general radiography cassettes, were also developed for mammography.

These film-screen systems were matched with dedicated mammography film processing units. These processing units produced film that had higher optical densities, blacks, and as such increased film/image contrast needed in mammography for breast imaging, as breasts have inherent low subject

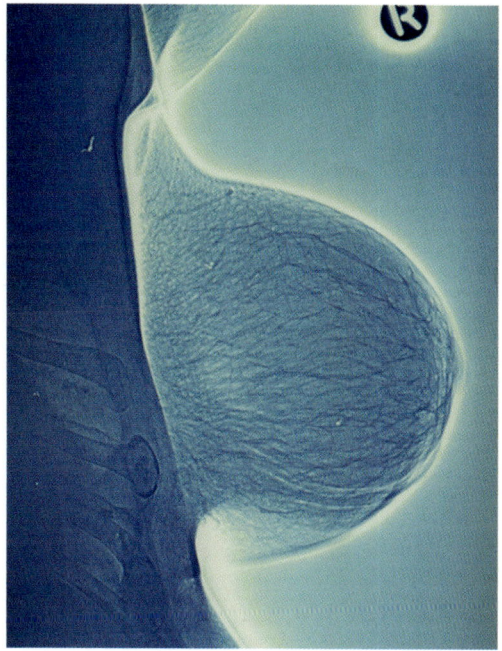

Figure 3.6 A xeromammography image. Note the inherent edge enhancement seen in the ribs and other object edges.

contrast. The main method to achieve higher optical densities in the film, compared to general radiography film processing, was by increasing the dwell time, the time the film spent in the developer solution.

Fuji Medical Systems introduced computed radiography (CR) systems in the 1980s. Not long after this, they developed a dedicated mammography CR system and digital imaging in mammography emerged. These mammography CR systems have increased spatial resolution, and the ability to visualize detail compared to general X-ray CR systems.

Mammography CR systems had the advantage of being able to quickly replace film-screen cassettes in existing mammography units. However, the main advantage, and it still is, in digital mammography systems is the so-called decoupling of the recording and viewing of images. In film-screen systems, the film was both the recording and viewing medium. The X-ray exposure in film-screen systems had to be precise and after processing, no adjustments in terms of image brightness and contrast nor other image alterations like edge enhancements could be made.

While CR is a digital modality, it can only capture one image on the image plate and then the image plate needs to be removed from the mammography unit and processed. A current breast imaging modality is tomosynthesis, see Chapter 4 for more information on this. Digital breast tomosynthesis requires multiple images to be captured within a few seconds and, as such, it is not compatible with CR.

Current Image Recording Systems

The current image capture method in mammography uses flat panel detectors (FPD). In FPD, X-ray photon energies are converted to electrical charges by one of two main processes. The first one indirectly converts photon energy to an electrical charge by first converting photon energy to multiple photons of visible light. The second of these directly converts photon energy to an electrical charge. The charges are then stored on and almost instantly readout using a thin film transistor (TFT) array. Figure 3.7 shows a diagrammatic representation of a TFT. The amount of charge stored and readout is proportional to the amount of X-ray photons that strike the FPD. The readout charge creates an electrical signal. Using an analog-to-digital conversion (ADC) process, an array of numbers or raw pixel values is created to form the image.

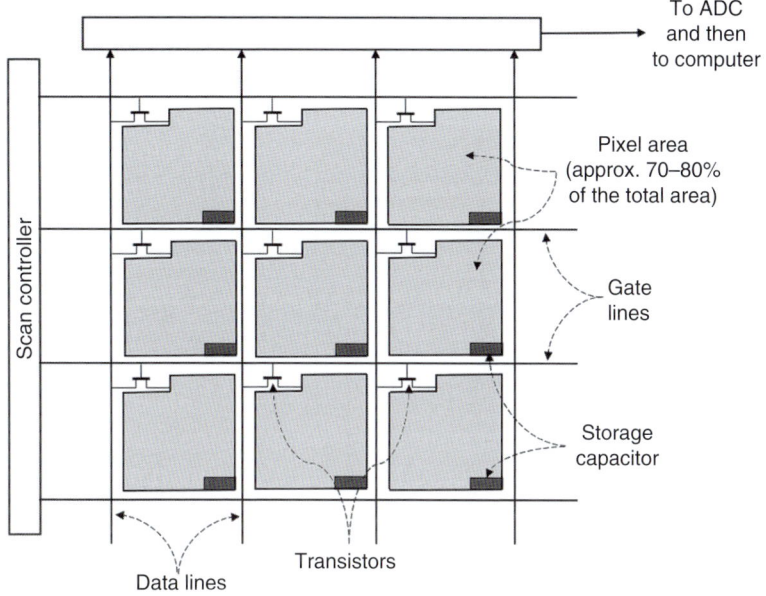

To ADC
and then
to computer

Pixel area
(approx. 70–80%
of the total area)

Scan controller

Gate
lines

Storage
capacitor

Transistors

Data lines

Figure 3.7 Diagram of a thin film array used in flat panel detectors.

In-Direct Flat Panel Detectors

In-direct flat panel detectors, used by some mammography unit manufacturers, use cesium iodide (CsI) to convert X-ray photons to light photons. Columns of CsI are laid over the top of amorphous silicon (a-Si) photodiodes. Following an interaction of the X-ray photon with a CsI crystal, energy from the X-ray photon is converted into multiple light photons. In mammography in-direct systems, the columns of CsI are needle-like structures to help reduce the spread of light in the CsI layer. The light in the CsI needle-like structures is directed toward an amorphous silicon (a-Si) thin film transistor. The light energy is then converted by the a-Si to an electrical charge and briefly stored in the thin film transistor. The TFT array charges are then readout to form the raw pixel values. Figure 3.8 compares this method and the direct conversion method.

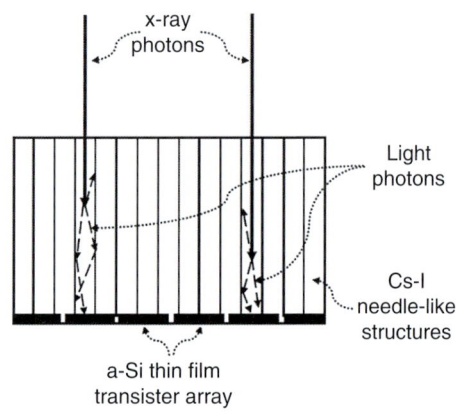

In-direct flat panel detector

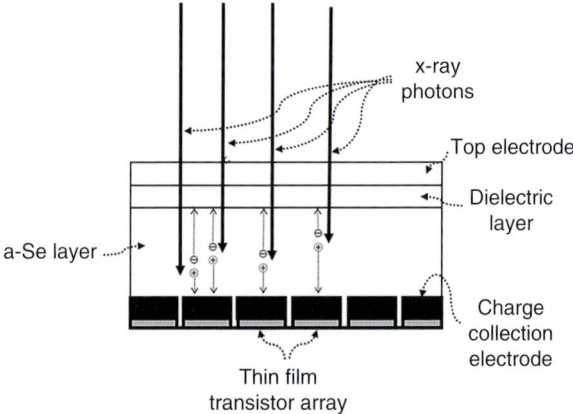

Direct flat panel detector

Figure 3.8 Flat panel detector processes. Left: The in-direct conversion method using cesium iodide (CsI) and amorphous silicon (a-Si) photodiodes. Right: The direct conversion method using amorphous selenium (a-Se).

Direct Flat Panel Detectors

Direct flat panel detectors, used by other mammography unit manufacturers, have an amorphous selenium (a-Se) layer where ionization event occurs when irradiated by X-rays. Positive and negative ions are created by the ionization event in this layer and are attracted in opposite directions by a voltage that is applied across the layer. Positive ions are attracted to the charge collection electrode which is situated over a thin film transistor. The charge in the TFT is proportional to the charge in the charge collection electrode, which is then readout to form the raw pixel values. Figure 3.8 compares this method and the in-direct conversion method.

Flat Panel Detectors Arrays

The flat panel detectors are typically 24×30 cm or 29×29 cm in dimension, as the largest size. Some manufacturers will enable the FPD to be swapped out for smaller FPDs such as 18×24 cm in size. Other manufacturers will turn off thin film transistors (TFTs) in their large FPD and collimate the X-ray beam, so the FPD is effectively 18×24 cm in size. This reduced area of 18×24 cm can also be shifted around inside the larger 24×30 FPD. Figure 3.9 shows an example of this where a shift of the 18×24 cm area to the left and right edges of the large FPD can improve patient positioning of the shoulder and arm for medial–lateral oblique projections.

The TFT sizes for mammography are in the range of 50 micrometers (μm) to 100 μm square with the most common size being 70–85 μm. The TFT size then sets the image pixel size and the number of pixels in each row and column of the image. Typical numbers of rows and columns of TFT's on the FPD are 2,400–2,500 rows by 3,000–3,500 columns.

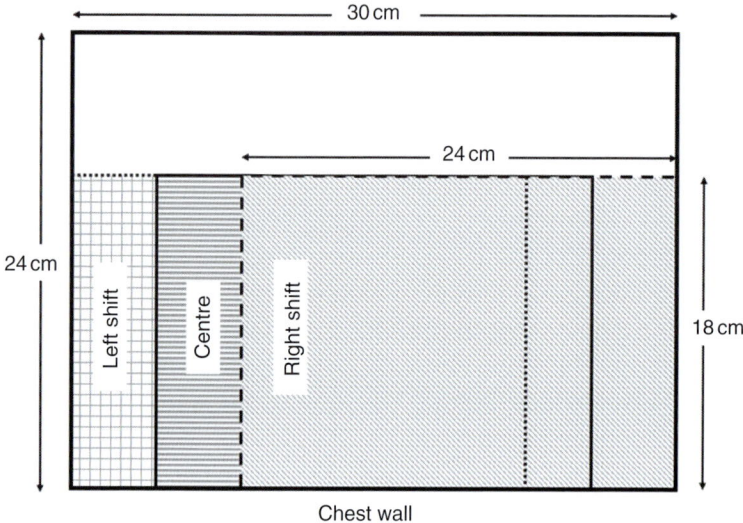

Figure 3.9 Shifting the 18×24 cm field area within the 24×30 cm flat panel detector to improve patient comfort in some projections.

The active area of each TFT typically only covers 70–80% of its area, see Figure 3.7. Around 20–30% in the TFT is the TFT's charge store and transistor areas. The spatial resolution that results from TFT of these sizes is 10 line-pairs per millimeter (lp/mm) for 50 μm TFT, 7.1 lp/mm for 70 μm size, and 5 lp/mm for 100 μm size.

The detective quantum efficiency (DQE) of an imaging system refers to the detectors' efficiency in converting the incident X-ray signal on the detector to an image signal. Formally, the DQE is the ratio of the detector output signal-to-noise ratio (SNR) squared and the detector input SNR squared at a given spatial frequency.

Both the in-direct a-Si and the direct a-Se flat panel detectors have overall better DQE than CR and film-screen imaging systems. This means to get the same output from these flat panel detectors as from CR and film-screen, a lower radiation input is needed, and hence reduced dose to the patient. The in-direct a-Si system does have a slightly higher DQE than the direct a-Se detectors.

Flat panel detectors also have and need a large dynamic range. The dynamic range is its ability to capture both a small number of photons incident on a single pixel and a very large number of incident photons without saturation. Saturation occurs when a detector is not able to capture any more photons and store more electrical charge prior to readout. If saturation occurs, potential information for the image is lost.

Image Generation

The electrical signal from the charge in the TFT that comes out of the flat panel detector is analog. In other words, the voltage generated by signal is infinitely variable between the minimum and maximum voltages. This information is not in a form that is suitable for a digital computer and must undergo analog-to-digital conversion (ADC). The large dynamic range of flat panel detectors need a large range of pixel values. In mammography, the raw images typically have a bit depth of 14 bits, which means there are 16,384 potential values to represent the number of X-ray photons striking each individual pixel. Importantly, 14 bits/16,384 potential values also mean that the infinitely varying voltage values are grouped into each digital value with less rounding error or less quantization error.

The raw digital values from the ADC process are used to create a raw image. This image is not ready for display on a monitor and viewing, see an example in Figure 3.9. This image is a positive image, typical of what is captured in all digital image recording devices, such as photography cameras and cell/mobile phones. In these devices, high intensities from the light are seen as bright areas or white. Medical imaging viewing is still based on X-ray film days when high intensities created high optical densities or blacks. Given the high dynamic range of the detector and the large bit depth if the image was viewed with a one-to-one look-up-table (LUT), the image would lack displayed perceived contrast and appear flat, as Figure 3.10. The histogram of the image in Figure 3.10 is shown in Figure 3.11. There are a very high number of pixel values near or at the value of 16,383 from the unattenuated X-rays striking the flat panel detector. The histogram also shows the relatively large spread of values from X-ray passing through the breast tissue and their low number compared to the background.

Pre-processing, a transformation process, is needed to convert the raw image to an image that is suitable for viewing and conforms to Digital Imaging and Communications in Medicine

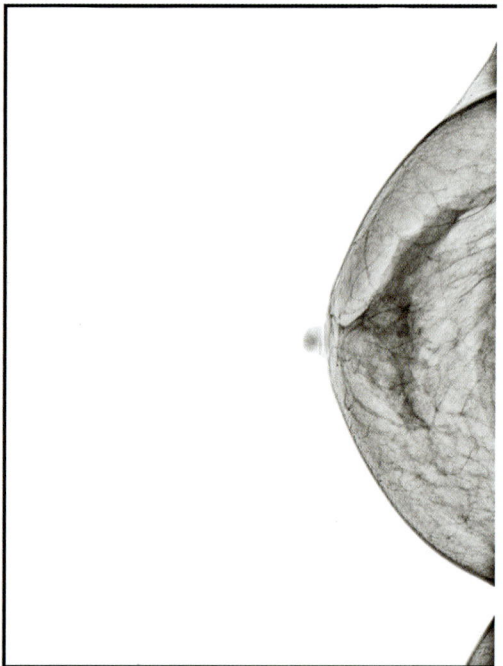

Figure 3.10 A raw image, a positive image, of the pixel values directly taken from the flat panel detector, with no pre-processing. This raw image has been converted to the image seen in Figure 1.1.
Source: With permission of BreastScreen ACT, Canberra, Australia.

Histogram–raw pixel values

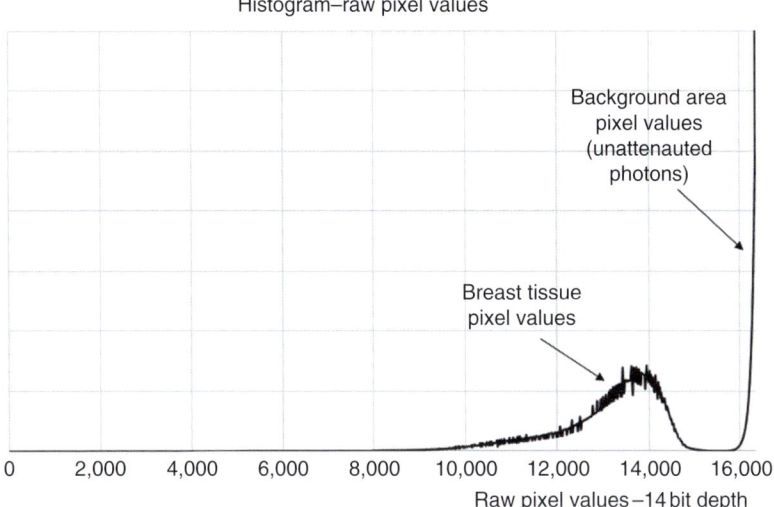

Figure 3.11 A histogram of the raw image seen in Figure 3.10. The X-axis scale is 14 bit depth/16,384 values with a large number of high values for the unattenuated background X-rays and a low number, in comparison, of pixel values from the breast tissue.

(DICOM) standards for storage, transmission, and viewing. The values of interest (VOI) LUT and transformation process are used to convert the raw image. In most systems, the raw image is stored for later processing if needed. The algorithm finds the minimum and maximum pixel values of the breast tissue, and in mammography, applies a sigmoid-shaped LUT to bring both the raw pixel values down to 12 bit/4,096 possible values and center the breast tissue values within that range. The left side of Figure 3.12 shows an example of the VOI sigmoid-shaped LUT curves with different slopes or window widths and different pixel value center locations or window levels or centers. The right side of Figure 3.12 shows the resultant image histogram. This image is then ready for storage and display. If the VOI LUT has worked correctly, the image will be optimized for displaying brightness and contrast.

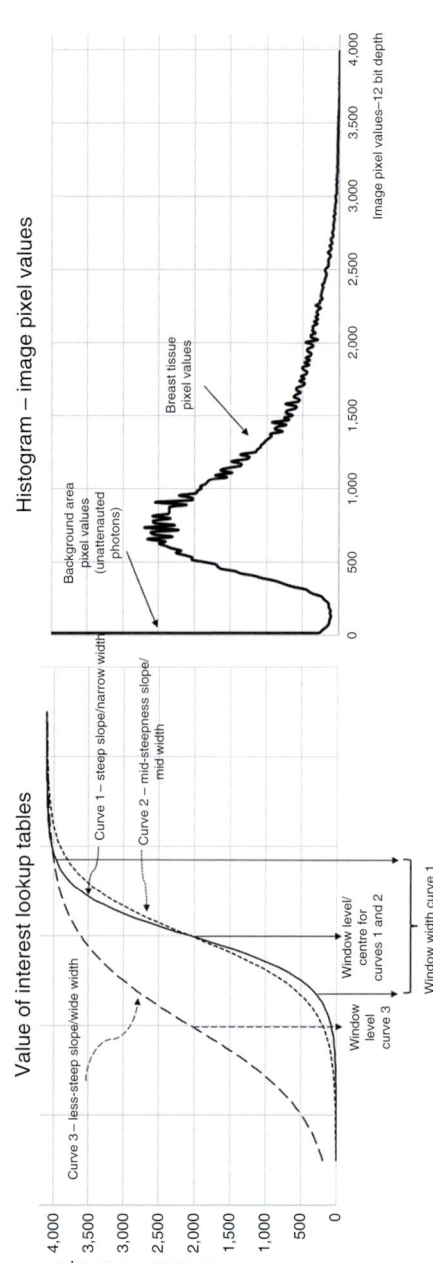

Figure 3.12 Left: Three sigmoid-shaped look-up-table (LUT) curves with different window widths (i.e. gradients/slopes) and different window levels or centers (i.e. the center value). Right: The resultant histogram from sigmoid-shaped values of interest (VOI) LUT curve applied to Figure 3.10 and its histogram is seen in Figure 3.11.

However, the displayed image brightness and contrast can be further adjusted to suit the viewer's needs, and this is achieved by using presentation LUTs, typically called window width (WW) to alter displayed contrast and window level (WL) to alter displayed brightness.

Part of the pre-processing algorithm can be a segmentation approach. There are significant differences between the pixel values of the breast tissue and the unattenuated X-ray beam, and as such, they create an edge that a computer algorithm can detect. The pixel values within the edges i.e. from within the breast tissue, are the only values then used to determine the shape and slope of the LUT.

DICOM Image File

Following the conversion process, the image is saved for storage and transfer and then displayed in DICOM format. DICOM format is used in all medical imaging and digital mammography to enable the standardization of medical imaging for storage on any compatible device, transfer between storage devices and display devices, and the display of the image and all the associated image data. The DICOM file header, also known as its metadata, is where the image information data is stored in the image file and has many types of data including:

- patient details such as
    - patient name, age, gender, etc.
    - referring physician, radiologist, mammographer/ mammography technologist
    - numbers that are unique to the examination and image
- image details such as
    - location in the file where the actual image data starts and ends
    - number of rows and columns
    - bit depth

- field size
- compressed breast thickness
- projection or view
- equipment details such as
    - focal spot size
    - target material
    - filter material
    - grid in or out
    - compression force
- exposure and dose information such as
    - kVp, mA, and time
    - SID
    - exposure control method
    - relative exposure/exposure index
    - calculated dose

Figure 3.13 shows a section of the DICOM header information with the tag number and name along with the attributes of that tag for this image.

The above method of digital mammography is often called 2D full-field digital mammography (FFDM) or just 2D mammography. So-called 3D mammography, more formally called digital breast tomosynthesis (DBT), is discussed in Chapter 4. DBT images viewed and displayed using similar processes to 2D FFDM images are discussed below.

Image Display

Once the image values underwent pre-processing/transformation processes, a DICOM-compliant image is created. During display, mammographic images undergo digital-to-analog conversion (DAC) for human visualization and perception. The monitor itself is the DAC tool that converts a digital value into a color or shade of gray that can be perceived by human observers.

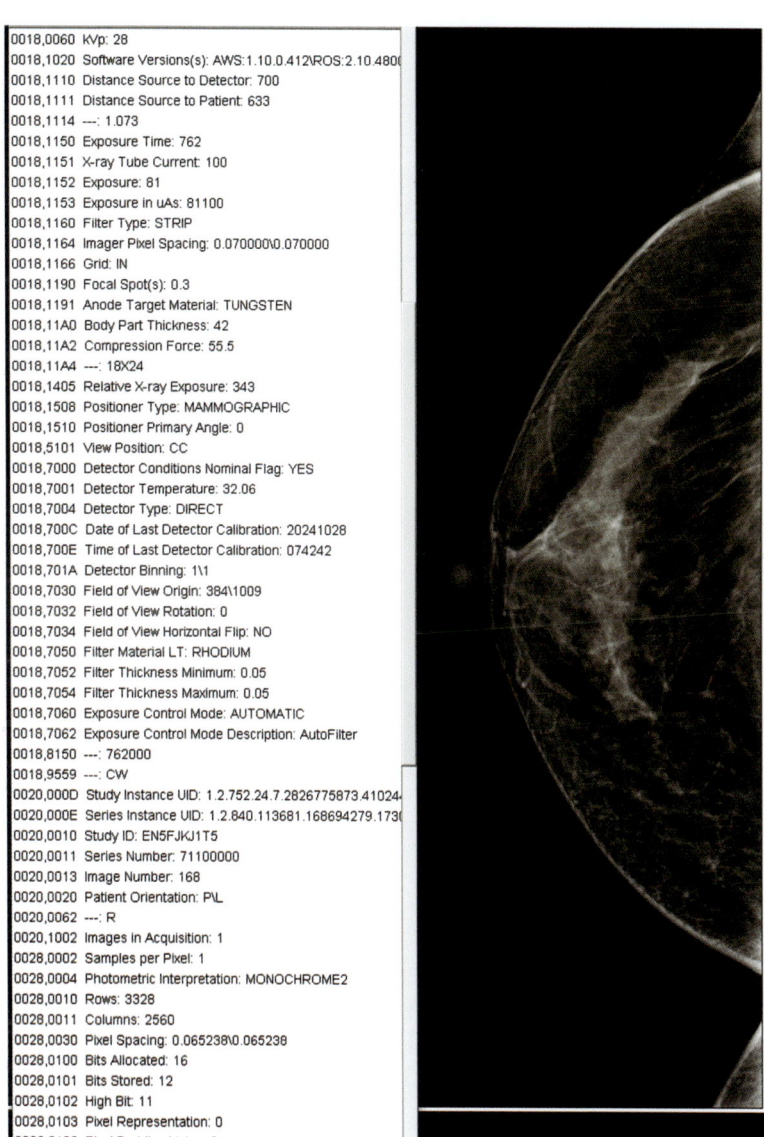

0018,0060	KVp: 28
0018,1020	Software Versions(s): AWS:1.10.0.412\ROS:2.10.480(
0018,1110	Distance Source to Detector: 700
0018,1111	Distance Source to Patient: 633
0018,1114	---: 1.073
0018,1150	Exposure Time: 762
0018,1151	X-ray Tube Current: 100
0018,1152	Exposure: 81
0018,1153	Exposure in uAs: 81100
0018,1160	Filter Type: STRIP
0018,1164	Imager Pixel Spacing: 0.070000\0.070000
0018,1166	Grid: IN
0018,1190	Focal Spot(s): 0.3
0018,1191	Anode Target Material: TUNGSTEN
0018,11A0	Body Part Thickness: 42
0018,11A2	Compression Force: 55.5
0018,11A4	---: 18X24
0018,1405	Relative X-ray Exposure: 343
0018,1508	Positioner Type: MAMMOGRAPHIC
0018,1510	Positioner Primary Angle: 0
0018,5101	View Position: CC
0018,7000	Detector Conditions Nominal Flag: YES
0018,7001	Detector Temperature: 32.06
0018,7004	Detector Type: DIRECT
0018,700C	Date of Last Detector Calibration: 20241028
0018,700E	Time of Last Detector Calibration: 074242
0018,701A	Detector Binning: 1\1
0018,7030	Field of View Origin: 384\1009
0018,7032	Field of View Rotation: 0
0018,7034	Field of View Horizontal Flip: NO
0018,7050	Filter Material LT: RHODIUM
0018,7052	Filter Thickness Minimum: 0.05
0018,7054	Filter Thickness Maximum: 0.05
0018,7060	Exposure Control Mode: AUTOMATIC
0018,7062	Exposure Control Mode Description: AutoFilter
0018,8150	---: 762000
0018,9559	---: CW
0020,000D	Study Instance UID: 1.2.752.24.7.2826775873.41024-
0020,000E	Series Instance UID: 1.2.840.113681.168694279.173(
0020,0010	Study ID: EN5FJKJ1T5
0020,0011	Series Number: 71100000
0020,0013	Image Number: 168
0020,0020	Patient Orientation: P\L
0020,0062	---: R
0020,1002	Images in Acquisition: 1
0028,0002	Samples per Pixel: 1
0028,0004	Photometric Interpretation: MONOCHROME2
0028,0010	Rows: 3328
0028,0011	Columns: 2560
0028,0030	Pixel Spacing: 0.065238\0.065238
0028,0100	Bits Allocated: 16
0028,0101	Bits Stored: 12
0028,0102	High Bit: 11
0028,0103	Pixel Representation: 0
0028,0120	Pixel Padding Value: 0

Figure 3.13 DICOM file attributes and associated data for this mammographic image. Source: With permission of BreastScreen ACT, Canberra, Australia.

Once the image is displayed on the monitor, many digital image processing (DIP) options are available for image enhancement and improved visualization. The main DIP processes are to

- alter brightness and contrast. Presentation LUTs, commonly known as WW/WL, that are similar to the transformation LUTs are used. In mammography, typically they are sigmoid-shaped LUTs, see Figure 3.12 for examples of sigmoid-shaped LUTs.

   To alter brightness, the WL is adjusted. Lowering the WL will make the image appear brighter and increasing the WL will make the image appear darker.

   To alter contrast, the WW is adjusted. To increase displayed image contrast, the WW is narrowed effectively by increasing the gradient angle or slope of the LUT. To decrease displayed image contrast, the WW is widened effectively decreasing the gradient angle or slope of the LUT.

- increase the displayed size of a section of or object in the breast image. Electronic zoom is used to enlarge or reduce the size of the displayed image. The main DIP processes used are bilinear and bicubic interpolation methods. Using these methods, variable zoom levels are available and tend to preserve the object's shape better.

- enhance edges in the image. Edge enhancement is commonly undertaken using a DIP process known as unsharp masking. The main inputs to control the unsharp mask process are the radius and the amount. A smaller radius will enhance smaller objects, and the amount adjusts the brightness and darkness of the edges. This can be done by either Fourier filters or spatial convolution kernels.

   Image smoothing, the opposite of edge enhancement, is rarely undertaken as this is essentially a blurring process.

■ Other image enhancement processes that are used are:

- ■ spatial frequency restoration and deblurring. These processes are often part of the preprocessing process and are used to enhance small objects in the image, such as microcalcification.

- ■ selective or adaptive noise reduction, to reduce image noise in selected regions of the image.

- ■ adaptive local contrast enhancement and multiscale processing. These methods are designed to reduce strong contrasts and image noise and enhance edges and subtle contrasts. The image tends to show more detail of fine structures and to be more homogenous visually from the center to the edges. Multiscale processes are usually a wavelet-based approach, not a frequency/Fourier approach.

- ■ global latitude reduction. Again, this process is often part of the preprocessing process discussed earlier and reduces the range of pixel values in the image so viewing and processing are undertaken easily.

Some image display and DIP applications are shown in Figure 3.14. A distance measurement is seen with two values. The value in brackets of 37.2 mm is the FPD pixel measurement of 34.6 mm multiplied by the calculated mean magnification factor (discussed in Chapter 2) of the breast. This factor depends on the compression plate, and hence breast thickness and height above the detector.

Display Monitors

The purpose of a monitor is to convert the pixel values to colors or shades of gray. This is the DAC process. Specific display monitors are needed to view mammography images. High-quality general radiology display monitors can be used; however, they

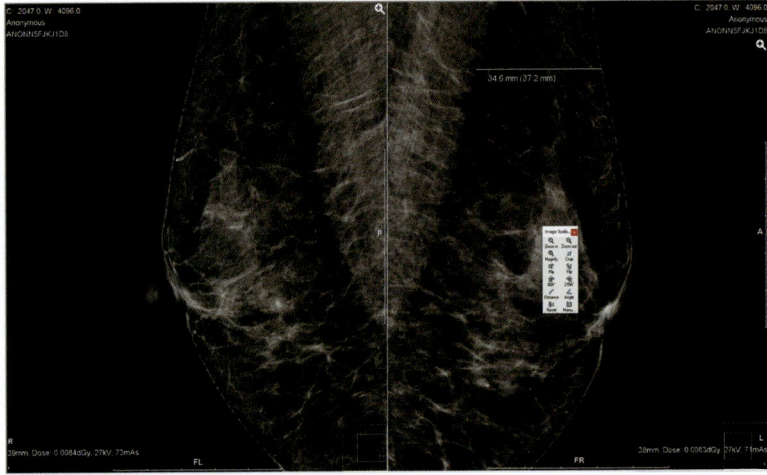

Figure 3.14 Side-by-side and magnified display of the right and left lateral oblique views of the breast. Also seen on the right side is a distance measurement and DIP tools. Source: With permission of BreastScreen ACT, Canberra, Australia.

are not the best option for mammography image viewing and interpretation. Several main differences exist between monitors used for mammography and those used for general radiology, and these are:

- the desire to display all individual image pixels on the monitor on a one-to-one basis.

  Mammography images have a large number of pixels. An image that is $2{,}400 \times 3{,}000$ has $7{,}200{,}000$ pixels or 7.2 mega-pixels (MP). To display all individual pixels, the monitor would need a (spatial) resolution of 7.2 MP.

  The screen resolution for mammography display monitors ranges between 5 and 12 MP. If a 5 MP monitor was used to display a 7.2 MP image, to display the entire image on the monitor, bilinear and bicubic interpolation methods would be needed to reduce the displayed size of the image, and as such one-to-one pixel display would not occur. However, 5 MP monitors are commonly used, and the level of image reduction is minimal and acceptable for high-quality display and interpretation of mammography image.

- small pixel sizes in the monitor. Typical pixel sizes are 0.1650×0.1650 mm and becoming smaller.
- the desire to compare left and right breast images side by side.

A single 12 MP monitor or two side-by-side 5 MP monitors are typically used to achieve side-by-side displays.

- the need to see strong blacks and bright whites.

A high brightness of the display increases the viewer's ability to visualize strong blacks and bright whites and as such their ability to visualize anatomy and pathology. Typical mammography monitors have a maximum luminance of 1,100 candela/square meter (cd/m^2) and some have up to 2,000 cd/m^2.

A high monitor contrast range is also needed to achieve this. Typical contrast ratios are around 850:1.

Mammography display monitors are normally black-and-white displays only, so color images cannot be displayed. The reasons for this are black and white monitor pixel sizes can be smaller, as each pixel area does not need three color light emitting diodes (LEDs) and higher brightness levels can also be achieved with black/white LEDs. Mammography images are only gray-scale images whereas other radiology images can be of color and as such color monitor monitors are needed in general radiology. If ultrasound, MRI, or other images are needed to assist with the diagnosis, often a second or third monitor with color display ability is used.

Some other considerations for mammography display monitors are:

- to comply with DICOM Standard, Part 14, Grayscale Standard Display Function, and various countries' standards such as the US Mammography Quality Standards Act (MQSA) standards for image presentation throughout the monitor's lifespan.
- to maintain a continuous level of brightness throughout the monitor's lifespan.
- be able to adjust light output to compensate for changes in ambient room lighting conditions.
- to have brightness consistent across the monitor display, that is, have brightness uniformity.

Conclusion

Acquiring and displaying a high-quality mammographic image is a complex process. Clinical mammography is more than just the understanding of the projections and required anatomy needed in a high-quality image. Mammographers/mammography technologists and breast clinicians should have a better understanding of the mammography principles, physics, and instrumentation. This is required so that optimization of the examination process can be undertaken, the radiation dose is minimized, and patient comfort and diagnosis from the acquired images are maximized.

Bibliography

Al Khalifah, K. H., Brindhaban, A. and Saeed, R. A. (2014). "Quality of images acquired with and without grid in digital mammography." *Radiological Physics and Technology* 7(1): 109–113.

Bushong, S. C. (2021). *Radiologic Science for Technologists*. Mosby.

Diffey, J. L. (2015). "A comparison of digital mammography detectors and emerging technology." *Radiography* 21(4): 315–323.

Fico, N., Di Grezia, G., Cuccurullo, V., Salvia, A. A. H., Iacomino, A., Sciarra, A. and Gatta, G. (2023). "Breast imaging physics in mammography (part I)." *Diagnostics (Basel)* 13(20): 3227.

Fico, N., Grezia, G. D., Cuccurullo, V., Salvia, A. A. H., Iacomino, A., Sciarra, A., La Forgia, D. and Gatta, G. (2023). "Breast imaging physics in mammography (part II)." *Diagnostics* 13(23): 3582.

Fredenberg, E., Willsher, P., Moa, E., Dance, D. R., Young, K. C. and Wallis, M. G. (2018). "Measurement of breast-tissue x-ray attenuation by spectral imaging: fresh and fixed normal and malignant tissue." *Physics in Medicine & Biology* 63(23): 235003.

Jouan, B. (1999). "Digital mammography performed with computed radiography technology." *European Journal of Radiology* 31(1): 18–24.

Leon, S. M., Brateman, L. F. and Wagner, L. K. (2014). "Characterization of scatter in digital mammography from physical measurements." *Medical Physics* 41(6 Part 1): 061901.

Nicosia, L., Gnocchi, G., Gorini, I., Venturini, M., Fontana, F., Pesapane, F., Abiuso, I., Bozzini, A. C., Pizzamiglio, M., Latronico, A., Abbate, F., Meneghetti, L., Battaglia, O., Pellegrino, G. and Cassano, E. (2023). "History of mammography: analysis of breast imaging diagnostic achievements over the last century." *Healthcare* 11(11): 1596.

Spahn, M. (2005). "Flat detectors and their clinical applications." *European Radiology* 15(9): 1934–1947.

Zhou, A., Tan, Q., White, G. L. and Davidson, R. (2021). "New anti-scatter grid design by optimization of strip thickness and height." *International Journal of Imaging Systems and Technology* 31(3): 1294–1299.

Zhou, A., Yin, Y., Tan, Q., White, G. L. and Davidson, R. (2020). "The determination of the optimal strip-thickness of anti-scatter grids for a given grid ratio and strip height." *International Journal of Imaging Systems and Technology* 30(4): 916–925.

4

Digital Breast Tomosynthesis and Advanced Techniques

Chapter at a Glance

- Introduction
- Stereotactic Digital Imaging Biopsies
- Contrast Enhance Mammography
- Digital Breast Tomosynthesis
- Photon Counting Mammography
- Bibliography

Introduction

Chapter 2 provided an overview of mammography instrumentation and looked at X-ray production and Chapter 3 looked at X-ray interaction in the breast, scatter control, and image formation. These two chapters covered topics in the so-called 2D mammography. This chapter looks at advanced mammographic techniques but still needs an understanding of the instrumentation, physics, and principles discussed in these earlier chapters.

Digital Mammography: Physics and Instrumentation, Second Edition. Rob Davidson.
© 2026 John Wiley & Sons Ltd. Published 2026 by John Wiley & Sons Ltd.

Stereotactic Digital Imaging Biopsies

Radiologists and other clinicians often need to confirm or eliminate the presence of pathology that is suspected from reviewing the mammogram images. One way of doing this is by inserting a needle in the mass and removing some tissue cells that can be examined by pathologists. To obtain the cells, a needle biopsy needs to be performed. From a 2D mammogram, the X and Y locations of any object, relative to the detector, can be easily determined. The image pixels have a specific size and using a computer, the X and Y locations of a point in the mass, as distance in millimeters, can be determined. What cannot be determined from a single 2D image is the Z distance or depth of the mass above the breast support or from the compression paddle. To determine this, Z-distance stereotactic methods are needed.

Digital stereotactic methods are based on very early radiology stereotactic methods where two images were taken of the patient. The focal point of the X-ray tube was offset left and right for each exposure from the usual centering point by a distance that is approximately equal to half the distance of a person's eyes, which is around 2–2.5 cm, each direction from the median sagittal plane of the body. The two resultant images were placed in a device where the radiologist could only see the left image with their left eye and the right image with their right eye. The radiologist's mind would merge the two images, and they would achieve depth perception and would "see" a 3D image from the two planar 2D images.

Digital stereotactic takes this method further and calculates the depth of the object under investigation so the radiologist can know the depth they need to insert the needle to obtain a biopsy sample of the mass. This requires

- ■ digital imaging as the distances in the images need to be calculated with a computer.

- the compression paddle, normally used in imaging, needs to be swapped out for a biopsy compression paddle that has holes in it for needle insertion.
- the method that involves taking at least two views, normally three views, being at angles of +10° to 15° from the vertical position, at the vertical position or 0° position, and at −10° to 15° from the vertical position. Figure 4.1, on the left, shows a diagrammatic representation of these positions with the breast under compression and an object (the square shape) at a depth in the breast.
- the resultant three images are shown on the right side of Figure 4.1. The object (the square shape) is seen to move in the images relative to the central line in the image depending on the angle of the X-ray tube and the object's/mass's location and depth in the breast during the exposure.
- the images are viewed, and the object/mass is marked.
- the computer that uses trigonometric calculations to determine the depth of the marked object/mass.
- the biopsy needle to be inserted at the determined X/Y location and to a depth in the breast that was calculated, and the breast is re-imaged to confirm the needle position in the object/mass.

Digital stereotactic biopsies can be performed using a standard mammography unit, with some additional software installed in the system and a dedicated biopsy compression paddle. There are however dedicated biopsy mammography units that allow the woman to lie prone on a table and the breast being biopsied is placed through a hole in the table. The imaging and biopsy are performed under the table. The advantage of such a dedicated unit is the woman's comfort during the procedures as the breast cannot be moved or the compression removed between the initial images and the reconfirmation of the needle's location in the object/mass.

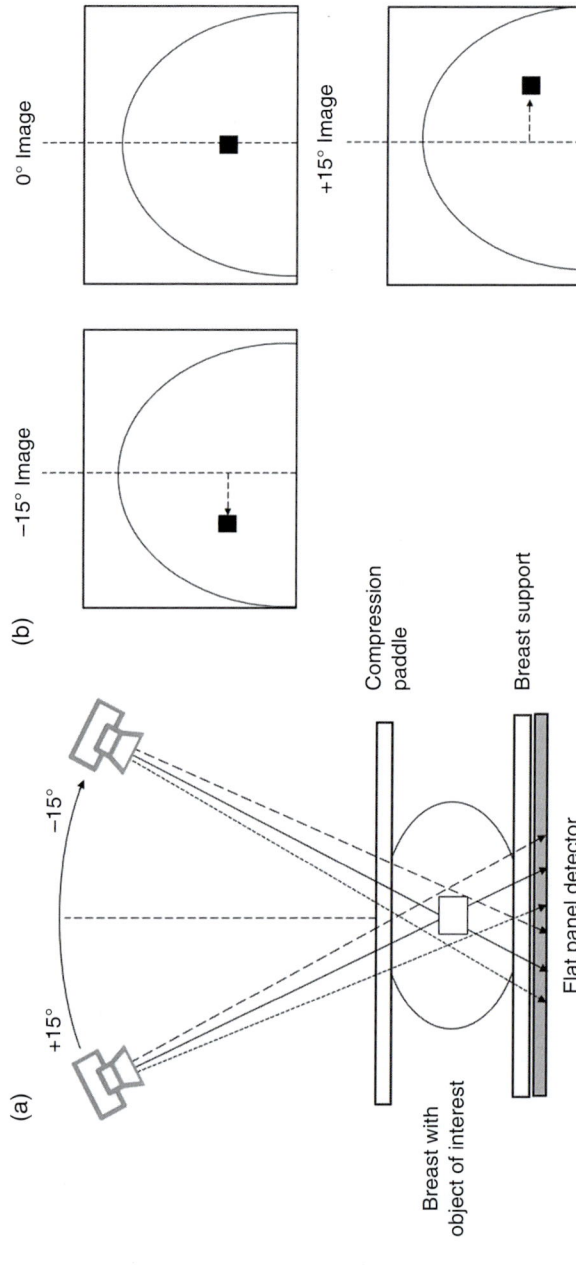

Figure 4.1 (a) Digital stereotactic methods showing the angle of the X-ray tube for the three images. (b) The resultant three images showing the object of interest, the square, moving in each image relative to the central line in the image.

Contrast Enhanced Mammography

Contrast enhanced mammography (CEM) is an emerging technique that has been shown to increase visualization of breast tumors. CEM is also known as contrast-enhanced dual-energy mammography and contrast-enhanced spectral mammography.

The basis of CEM imaging is the use of low-osmolarity iodine-based contrast material injected into the patient. Without moving the patient between exposures, two images per breast projection are acquired: a low X-ray energy beam image and a high-energy X-ray beam image.

The X-ray exposures are timed to allow for the iodinated contrast material to diffuse within tumor tissue. This is around 2–2.5 minutes after the contrast injection to maximize tumor visualization. As iodinated contrast material is rapidly excreted from the body, imaging needs to be completed within 8–10 minutes after the contrast injection.

As discussed in Chapter 2, the energy of the X-ray beam is controlled by the voltage applied across the X-ray tube (the kVp setting) and the target/filter combination is selected. The low-energy image has an exposure setting that would be used for that woman's breast, for example, 25–34 kVp and the recommended target/filter combination for that breast thickness and expected composition is selected. The high-energy image setting is dependent on the unit but typical kVp settings are 45–49 kVp and target/filter combinations of tungsten (W)/silver (Ag) or titanium (Ti) and molybdenum (Mo) or rhodium (Rh) with both aluminum (Al) and Rh filter materials.

The high-energy image is used to create an iodine image that shows areas of contrast enhancement. The K-edge of iodine is 33.2 keV. Using a beam that has photon energies above this value increases the amount of attenuation from iodine-filled structures and as a result, improves image contrast. Given the high energy used to create this image, the unprocessed image has very low image contrast. The high-energy image is digitally processed with the low-energy image to create a recombined image. This image is created by subtracting the low-energy image from the high-energy image. This process suppresses the background breast tissue and highlights areas where iodine is in the tissue. Both the low-energy and recombined images are viewed and reported by the radiologist.

CEM imaging has been shown to be most effective when the breast tissue is dense; the 2D and 3D imaging methods have lower sensitivity and specificity, measures of the imaging's diagnostic accuracy, when breast tissue is dense.

Digital Breast Tomosynthesis

Digital breast tomosynthesis (DBT) or so-called 3D breast imaging was developed late in the first decade of the 2000s and was approved for use in the United States by the US Food and Drug Administration (FDA) in 2011 and by authorities in many other countries. Studies have shown DBT to be superior to full-field digital mammography (FFDM) or 2D mammography for the early detection of breast cancer.

DBT produces a stack of 2D image slices, a pseudo-three-dimensional (psuedo-3D) image set, of the breast by taking multiple low-dose images or projections along an arc over the breast for each DBT examination. These resultant images/projections are then reconstructed to create a series of thin slices of the breast parallel to the flat panel detector (FPD). DBT is based on the principle of tomography that was used in general radiographic imaging prior to the advent and popular use of computed tomography (CT). A diagram of the tomography principles is shown in Figure 4.2.

In tomography, the X-ray exposure is commenced, and the tube and image plate move in synchronization but in opposite directions to each other during a long, several seconds, exposure. The movement is essentially an arc between the tube and the

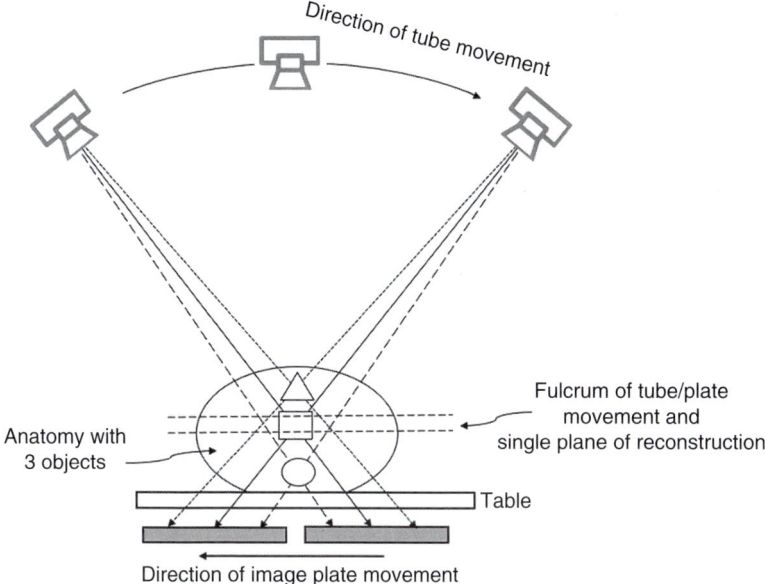

Figure 4.2 Tomography principles. The X-ray tube and image plate move in synchronization and opposite directions during a single long X-ray exposure to create a single image per exposure from the anatomy at the level of the fulcrum.

image plate with the fulcrum, or a pivot location, at the center. The image of the anatomy, above or below the fulcrum, will move across the plate during the exposure blurring the images of that anatomy. The image of the anatomy at the fulcrum essentially stays stationary relative to the image plate as it moves and as such is in focus. The anatomy at the fulcrum is visualized in the image while the anatomy above and below is blurred and not visualized. A single image of that slice of the anatomy is created. The greater the angle of the arc, the thinner the slice. To create images of other areas of anatomy, the patient's anatomy must be raised or lowered through the fulcrum and a new image is created. To create image slices of all the anatomy, multiple images, hence exposures of X-rays, are needed

Digital breast tomosynthesis principles are similar to tomography; however, there are some significant differences. Figure 4.3 shows a diagrammatic representation of the DBT principles. The first difference is that the FPD remains stationary while the X-ray tube moves during the several seconds of exposure. During the exposure, the FPD records and creates multiple images from different angles of the X-ray tube in the arc known as projections. The number of projects depends on the angle of the arc and varies between 9 and 25 projections. These projects are captured in one of two ways. The most common is that the X-ray beam is continually turned on during the movement of the X-ray tube and the FPD is turned on and off rapidly, known as gating, for a time of around 10 ms per capture. Such a short capture time stops blur in the projection images from X-ray tube movement. In the other method, the X-ray beam rapidly

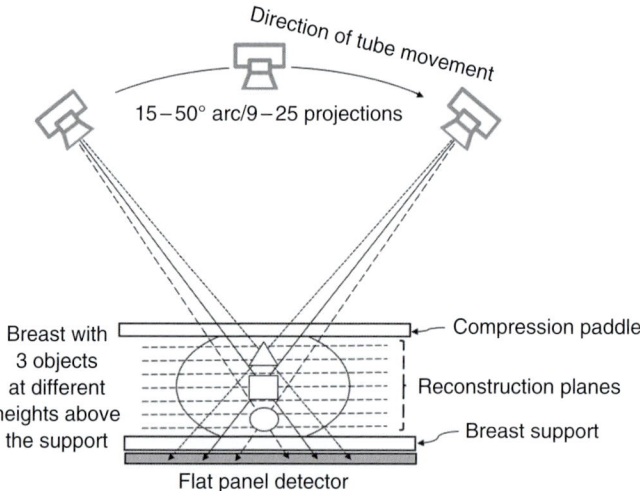

Figure 4.3 Digital breast tomosynthesis principles. The X-ray tube moves in 15–50° arc and the flat panel detector remains stationary during the few seconds of X-ray exposure to create multiple images per a single exposure from the anatomy at multiple levels in the breast.

turned on and off during the capture of the projections. This method is known as step and shoot. Overall exposure and tube movement times vary between 4 and 22 seconds depending on the manufacturers.

One mammography unit manufacturer, during the X-ray tube movement and exposure, angles FPD $\pm 2.1°$ in order to better align the FPD with the X-ray tube. All other manufacturers kept the FPD stationary.

The next difference between DBT and tomography is in DBT multiple images that are created during a single movement of the X-ray tube and during the exposure. Similar to CT, the projections, in this case, projection images, are used to create multiple images. Each final reconstructed image represents a small thickness of the breast tissue, typically one to a few millimeters thick, and at different heights above the breast support.

The process of reconstructing the images from the projection images is shown in Figure 4.4. Each of the seven projections is obtained at a different angle of the X-ray tube. As such, the image of the three objects, a circle, a square, and a triangle, in each projection image move relative to each other in each of the projection images.

The methods used to reconstruct the images from the projection images are all mathematical methods as pixel values are numbers. The easiest method to explain is the simple back projection or "shift and add" method and is shown in Figure 4.4.

In Figure 4.4b, the projections are not offset relative to each other projection. In this case, the projection images of the square object align with each other and the circle and triangle do not align. Mathematical casting rays are projected down the reconstructed image matrix. The pixel values along the rays are summed together to form the values in the reconstructed image. In this case, the aligned images of the square objects in each projection will sum together in the reconstructed image; however, the circle and triangle will not sum together as they are in different locations in each projection and essentially will be

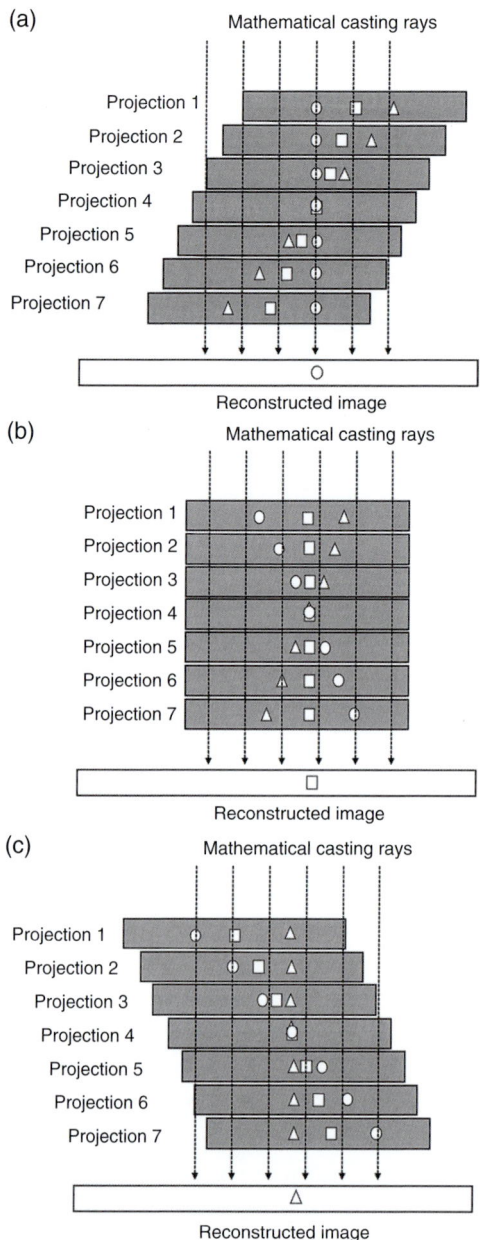

Figure 4.4 Digital breast tomosynthesis reconstruction process of simple back projection or "add and shift." The seven projections are seen side on and show the different locations of the objects relative to each other, caused by different X-ray tube angles for each projection.

blurred in the reconstructed image. The resultant reconstructed image is a 2D slice from the middle of the breast.

In Figure 4.4a, the projections have been shifted relative to each other. With this amount of shift, the images of the circle are aligned in each projection and added together, however, the square and triangle do not align and are not summed together in this reconstructed image. This reconstructed image is a slice from the anatomy of the breast closer to the breast support. Another shift in the projections is shown in Figure 4.4c. Here the images of the triangle align and are added together in the reconstructed image. This reconstructed image is a slice from the anatomy of the breast closer to the top of the breast or to the compression paddle.

The outcome of this reconstruction process is that multiple thin images are created that are parallel to breast support at different heights above the support. In this example, images are reconstructed with three of the reconstructed images showing the circle, the square, and the triangle only while blurring the other objects.

The mathematical processes that are and can be used in DBT image reconstruction are:

- filtered back projection, the most commonly used method,
- iterative reconstruction method,
- algebraic reconstruction technique (ART), and
- maximum-likelihood expectation maximization.

The number of reconstructed images produced is determined by the height of the compression paddle, and hence the breast thickness, above the breast support. Depending on the manufacturer, a typical slice thickness produced represents approximately 1 mm of breast tissue. The thickness depends primarily on the angle of the arc. There is also a distance between slice height locations, which ranges from 0.5 to 1.0 mm.

A measure of how well the slice represents the anatomy or objects is called the slice-sensitivity profile (SSP). This is the z-resolution of the image slices resulting from the angle of the arc and the reconstruction process.

The size of the pixels in the DBT reconstructed image slices, the in-plane resolution of the image, is typically similar to or slightly larger than the size of the pixels in the same manufacturer's 2D images. The pixels are square, and sizes range from 85 to 140 μm (0.085 to 0.14 mm) square.

A comparison between 2D and DBT mediolateral oblique images of the same woman is shown in Figure 4.5.

(a) (b)

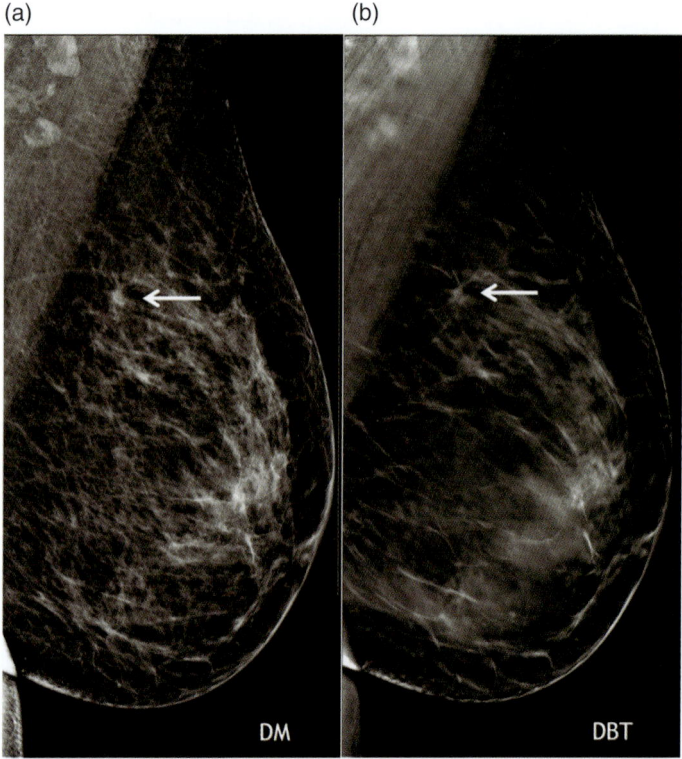

Figure 4.5 A 2D mammogram (a) and digital breast tomosynthesis (b) mediolateral oblique images of the same woman. A small spiculated mass is seen (arrow).
Source: With permission of Gao et al., (2021) / Radiological Society of North America.

Similar to CT, the reconstructed images can be mathematically stacked back together, and further images can be created. However, in CT, these images would represent, for example, sagittal or coronal planes or three-dimensional (3D) representations of the anatomy. In DBT, the stacking and further reconstruction are used to create an image similar to a 2D image of the breast. This resulting image has various names from different manufacturers, for example, C-view, V-preview, and insight-2D. These images do not have the same high level of image quality as 2D images acquired using normal mammographic techniques, and they should not be used to replace these images for diagnostic purposes.

Clinically, the current literature suggests that a breast imaging examination using DBT has higher diagnostic accuracy than FFDM, especially for women with dense breasts. The difference between DBT and FFDM diagnostic accuracy and detection of micro-calcifications for women with non-dense breasts is similar. However, for a single projection, FFDM has a lower dose than DBT (more details on this are in Chapter 5).

Photon-Counting Mammography

Photon-counting mammography (PCM) is the latest development in breast imaging. While it has yet to be fully accepted as the preferred breast imaging method and yet to be approved for use in some countries, it does have some advantages over the standard flat-panel detector method in digital mammography.

In FFDM, and other X-ray imaging methods using FPDs, the X-ray photons that are incident on each of the FPD's pixel areas are summed, or integrated, together at the end of the X-ray exposure and are readout as an amount of charge from the thin-film transistor. The amount of charge undergoes analog-to-digital conversion (ADC) to create a digital value (see Chapter 3 for more detail). In PCM, the incident individual X-ray photons are detected using silicon strip detectors and are counted.

The photons are counted within a range of energies called energy windows or bins. There are typically only a small number of energy windows/bins, two or four; however, low photon energies from scatter radiation typically fall below the lowest energy window/bin and as such are not counted. This then acts as a scatter or noise reduction method. A further scatter reduction method in PCM is the image capture method using a slit-scanning technique. The PCM detector is a small number of silicon strips, and these are scanned across the X-ray field. Scatter not along the strip line direction is not detected and does not contribute to the image.

The main advantage of PCM is the reduced radiation dose compared to conventional mammography. Other advantages are

- improved contrast-to-noise ratio due to the use of the energy windows/bins.
- ability to better determine breast composition and possibly characterize breast lesions.
- contrast-enhanced mammography techniques, using a wider range of k-edge-based contrast agents, will potentially further improve diagnosis.
- tomosynthesis using photon counting methods is being evaluated with potential dose reductions, however, technical difficulties due to the slit-scanning methods still exist.

Breast Computed Tomography

Breast computed tomography (BCT) has been in use clinically for several decades. These units use X-ray technology and are based on cone beam geometry, that is, the detector is an FPD, not rows of detectors that are used in conventional CT. The detectors are typically made of the same materials as used in in-direct amorphous silicon (aSi) FPD, which was discussed in Chapter 3.

Advantages/disadvantages of BCT are:

- It has high contrast resolution, similar to general CT. BCT has the highest contrast resolution of all breast X-ray imaging modalities.
- However, the spatial resolution of BCT in the 2D direction (the in-plane resolution of CT) is significantly less than FFDM and DBT.
- BCT slice thickness, or its so-called cross-plane resolution is approximately one-fifth the thickness of a DBT slice.
- X-ray exposure times are longer than FFDM but similar to DBT.
- Radiation dose of BCT is similar to an FFDM
- Some literature states that breast tissue may be missed near the chest wall using CT, however, others state that the anatomical coverage of the breast tissue is the same.

Clinically, while the literature typically states improved detections of lesions and similar detection of calcifications, BCT is not as widely used as FFDM and DBT.

Conclusions

Breast image capture methods have been and are changing. Digital breast mammography, supported by DBT, still remains the gold standard in breast imaging and breast cancer detection. Any new breast imaging method must be able to improve lesion detectability, and then diagnose or maintain diagnostic levels, and significantly reduce radiation dose and risk to the patients.

Other breast image methods exist that are not X-ray based. The most commonly used modalities are ultrasound and magnetic resonance imaging (MRI) with others such as thermography also being used. They complement X-ray-based image methods and can assist in improving the diagnosis for the woman; however, they are not discussed in this book.

Bibliography

Aminololama-Shakeri, S. and Boone, J. M. (2024). "Dedicated breast CT: getting ready for prime time." *Journal of Breast Imaging* 6(5): 465–475.

Barber, W. C., Wessel, J. C., Malakhov, N., Wawrzyniak, G., Hartsough, N. E., Nœss-Ulseth, E. and Iwanczyk, J. S. (2015). Photon counting systems for breast imaging. *2015 IEEE Nuclear Science Symposium and Medical Imaging Conference (NSS/MIC).*

Bushong, S. C. (2021). *Radiologic Science for Technologists.* Mosby.

Cole, E. B., Toledano, A. Y., Lundqvist, M. and Pisano, E. D. (2012). "Comparison of radiologist performance with photon-counting full-field digital mammography to conventional full-field digital mammography." *Academic Radiology* 19(8): 916–922.

Davidson, R., Al Khalifah, K. and Zhou, A. (2022). "Variation in digital breast tomosynthesis image quality at differing heights above the detector." *Journal of Medical Radiation Sciences* 69(2): 174–181.

Dhamija, E., Gulati, M., Deo, S. V. S., Gogia, A. and Hari, S. (2021). "Digital breast tomosynthesis: an overview." *Indian Journal of Surgical Oncology* 12(2): 315–329.

Gao, Y., Moy, L. and Heller, S. L. (2021). "Digital breast tomosynthesis: update on technology, evidence, and clinical practice." *RadioGraphics* 41(2): 321–337.

Hernandez, A. M., Seibert, J. A., Nosratieh, A. and Boone, J. M. (2017). "Generation and analysis of clinically relevant breast imaging x-ray spectra." *Medical Physics* 44(6): 2148–2160.

Jochelson, M. S. and Lobbes, M. B. I. (2021). "Contrast-enhanced mammography: state of the art." *Radiology* 299(1): 36–48.

Johansson, H., von Tiedemann, M., Erhard, K., Heese, H., Ding, H., Molloi, S. and Fredenberg, E. (2017). "Breast-density measurement using photon-counting spectral mammography." *Medical Physics* 44(7): 3579–3593.

Kopans, D. B. (2014). "Digital breast tomosynthesis from concept to clinical care." *American Journal of Roentgenology* 202(2): 299–308.

Nelson, J. S., Wells, J. R., Baker, J. A. and Samei, E. (2016). "How does c-view image quality compare with conventional 2D FFDM?" *Medical Physics* 43(5): 2538–2547.

Nicosia, L., Gnocchi, G., Gorini, I., Venturini, M., Fontana, F., Pesapane, F., Abiuso, I., Bozzini, A. C., Pizzamiglio, M., Latronico, A., Abbate, F., Meneghetti, L., Battaglia, O., Pellegrino, G. and Cassano, E. (2023). "History of mammography: analysis of breast imaging diagnostic achievements over the last century." *Health* 11(11): 1596.

O'Connell, A., Conover, D. L., Zhang, Y., Seifert, P., Logan-Young, W., Lin, C.-F. L., Sahler, L. and Ning, R. (2010). "Cone-beam CT for breast imaging: radiation dose, breast coverage, and image quality." *American Journal of Roentgenology* 195(2): 496–509.

O'Connell, A. M., Karellas, A. and Vedantham, S. (2014). "The potential role of dedicated 3D breast CT as a diagnostic tool: review and early clinical examples." *The Breast Journal* 20(6): 592–605.

Seeram, E. (2023). *Computed Tomography: Physical Principles, Patient Care, Clinical Applications and Quality Control.* Maryland Heights, Missouri, Elsevier.

Tirada, N., Li, G., Dreizin, D., Robinson, L., Khorjekar, G., Dromi, S. and Ernst, T. (2019). "Digital breast tomosynthesis: physics, artifacts, and quality control considerations." *RadioGraphics* 39(2): 413–426.

5

Radiation Exposure and Patient Dose

Chapter at a Glance

- Introduction
- Basic Concepts of Radiation Measurement
  - Radiation Exposure
  - Radiation Dose
  - Equivalent Dose
  - Effective Dose
  - Mean Glandular Dose
  - Calculating Mean Glandular Dose
  - Typical Doses
- Putting Radiation Dose in Perspective
  - Health Risks of Radiation
  - Shielding During Mammography Examination
  - Putting It All Together
- Bibliography

Digital Mammography: Physics and Instrumentation, Second Edition.
Rob Davidson.
© 2026 John Wiley & Sons Ltd. Published 2026 by John Wiley & Sons Ltd.

Introduction

As discussed in Chapter 2, X-rays are electromagnetic radiation, a type of *light*, that can pass through soft tissues. This property is associated with X-rays having very small wavelengths (approximately $1 \text{Å} = 0.1 \text{nm} = 10^{-10} \text{m}$). Planck's equation states that this small wavelength must be accompanied by high-photon energy:

$$E = hf \text{ or } E = \frac{hc}{\lambda}$$

where

E is the photon energy;
h is Planck's constant $= 6.626 \times 10^{-34} \text{J/Hz}$ (or 4.14×10^{-15} eV.s);
f is the frequency in Hertz (Hz);
c is the speed of light $= 3 \times 10^8$ m/s;
λ is the wavelength in meters;
hc is approximately 1.24×10^8 eV.m.

In the case of mammographic X-rays, a typical beam's average photon energy is approximately 18 keV. This energy is more than sufficient to dislodge electrons from their atoms, thus X-rays are referred to as *ionizing radiation*. There are two main types of effects caused by the X-ray photons or the highly energetic electrons ejected by ionizing radiation. These are

- Direct effects, where the initial ionization event occurs within a cell of a molecule, for example, in a DNA chain
- Indirect effects, where the initial ionization event occurs within a water molecule. These events can create free radicals, such as hydroxyl radicals (OH), which are chemically active. Approximately 60–70% of DNA damage is caused by hydroxyl radicals.

The deleterious effects following direct and indirect effects of ionization events are:

- Breaking molecular bonds:
  - Can cause mutations in DNA

- Can induce cancer in normal tissue
- Can cause birth defects in the case of fetal exposure
- Cross-linking (attaching) proteins
- Damaging normal tissue (high doses of radiation are needed for this to occur)
    - Skin erythema (may occur in mammography if filtration is absent)
    - Cataracts (high doses of radiation are needed for this to occur)

There is, once again, a trade-off. The same radiation that is valuable for diagnosing disease has the potential, albeit a small chance, of *causing* disease. The risks and benefits of radiation delivery must be carefully balanced. This concept is especially important for breast cancer screening, in which radiation is delivered to a large number of asymptomatic women. Before considering the risks and benefits of radiation, some basic descriptors of radiation delivery are defined.

Basic Concepts of Radiation Measurement

The X-ray beam that is delivered to a patient can be described in two ways, which will now be defined along with the units of measurement.

Radiation Exposure

Radiation exposure is a measure of the *quantity* of X-rays, the number of photons delivered, which for a typical mammographic exposure, is approximately 100,000,000,000,000,000,000 (10^{20}).

- Radiation exposure can be measured directly using an exposure meter, also referred to as a dosimeter (actually a misnomer) or ion chamber.
- Exposure measurement takes advantage of ionization that occurs as X-rays pass through air. The electrons and positive ions created by the X-rays are collected in the ion chamber.

- The recommended unit of radiation exposure is coulombs/kilogram (C/kg). This is an SI (the international system) unit. This measurement means that a certain quantity of electrical charge, C, is produced when 1 kg of air (approximately 1 cubic meter) is irradiated by X-rays.
- The non-SI unit of exposure measurement is the roentgen (R). The C/kg replaced R in 1975 and 1 R is equal to 2.58×10^{-4} C/kg.
- 1 C/kg (or 3,876 R) is an extremely large X-ray exposure.

Exposure is a useful, important X-ray measurement because it is easy to perform. Anyone with an exposure meter having a proper response to low-energy X-rays can make mammography exposure measurements that can be compared with exposure measurements made by any other investigator.

Radiation Dose

Although the measurement of exposure is convenient, it does not answer the important question, "What is the risk to the patient from this radiation?" Radiation risk and the potential for damage are related to the energy that is deposited by the X-rays as they interact with and are absorbed by the tissue. Essential concepts, definitions, and methodology for calculating radiation dose are as follows:

- Absorbed radiation dose (D) is defined as the energy deposited per unit mass by the delivery of an X-ray exposure.
- The unit used for the absorbed dose is gray (Gy), an SI unit. One gray equals 1 J of energy deposited in a kilogram of tissue.
- The non-SI unit of absorbed radiation dose is rad (**r**adiation **a**bsorbed **d**ose). A gray equals 100 rad (1 Gy = 100 rad).

■ Absorbed radiation dose is difficult to measure directly. However, dosimeters (exposure meters/ion chambers) can be calibrated to show dose in Gy, so the difference between the entrance dose (X-ray measurements on the surface of the breast) and the exit dose (X-ray measurements exiting the breast) is a measure of the breast's (or other objects) absorbed dose.

■ As it is not practical, nor clinically advisable, to use dosimeters during mammography examinations, so patient radiation dose must be calculated.

Equivalent Dose

Absorbed radiation dose is a measure of the energy deposited by radiation in tissue. Equivalent dose (H) is a related quantity that considers the *biologic effects* that result from the absorbed dose.

■ The unit for equivalent dose is the sievert (Sv), an SI unit.
■ The non-SI unit for equivalent dose is the rem (rad equivalent man). $1\,\mathrm{Sv} = 100\,\mathrm{rem}$.
■ The equivalent dose (Sv) is calculated by multiplying the absorbed dose, D, in Gy, by a radiation-weighting factor (w_R) for the radiation being used.
  ■ $H = D \times w_R$
  ■ The weighting factor (w_R) for X-rays is 1, which means that for mammography, $1\,\mathrm{Gy} = 1\,\mathrm{Sv}$.
  ■ Other weighting factors, though not used in mammography, are
    ■ gamma radiation and beta particles are 1
    ■ protons are 2
    ■ alpha particles are 20
    ■ neutrons (a function of their energy) are between 5 and 20
■ Personnel dosimeter exposures are usually reported as the dose equivalent (Sv) received.

Effective Dose

As some organs or body parts are more sensitive to ionizing radiation than others, the effective dose ϵ is used as a dose-reporting scheme that can calculate the overall effect on the whole body when the whole body is not irradiated or when more than one tissue or organ is irradiated. It can be used for comparing the "dose" in one medical imaging examination, for example, a mammogram, to the "dose" in another medical imaging examination, for example, a CT scan of the head.

- Tissue-weighting factors (w_T) are assigned to specific tissues or organs and the whole body tissue weighting factors add up to 1.0 (or 100%). The tissue weighting factors are set out in table 3 of the 2007 International Commission on Radiological Protection (ICRP) Publication 103.
- The tissue-weighting factor for breast tissue is 0.12 (or 12% of the whole body). Other w_T are shown in Table 5.1. Note that breasts are equally the most radiosensitive human organ.

Table 5.1 Tissue Weighting Factors (w_T) of Organs/Body Parts as Some Organs or Tissues Are More Radiosensitive Than Others. The Whole Body = 1.0 or 100%.

Tissue	Weighting	Tissue	Weighting
Breast	**0.12**	Gonads	0.08
Lung	0.12	Bladder	0.04
Colon	0.12	Esophagus	0.04
Stomach	0.12	Liver	0.04
Red bone-marrow	0.12	Thyroid	0.04
Remainder of the body	0.12	Bone surface, brain, salivary glands, skin (each)	0.01

Source: Adapted from ICRP Publication 103, 2007, Recommendations of the International Commission on Radiological Protection

- Example of effective dose calculation:
    - A woman receives a total absorbed dose to both her breasts during a mammogram (X-rays) of 3 mGy:

$$\text{effective dose, } E_{\text{Breasts}} = D_{\text{Breasts}} \times w_{R(X-ray)} \times w_{T(\text{Breasts})}$$
$$= 3 \times 1 \times 0.12$$
$$\text{effective dose} = 0.36 \, \text{mSv}$$

Mean Glandular Dose

Currently, mammography is the only radiographic procedure for which there is universal agreement on how radiation dose should be calculated and reported. Dose specification and reporting in mammography should always be in terms of mean glandular dose (D_g).

- Mean glandular dose is the same as *average glandular dose.*
- Calculated using the following scheme:
    - Radiation *exposure* to the breast is multiplied by an *exposure-to-dose conversion factor* that depends on:
        - Half-value layer (effective X-ray beam energy), which is dependent on
            - peak kilovolts (kVp)
            - target/anode and filter materials
        - Breast thickness
        - Breast tissue type

Calculating Mean Glandular Dose

If there is ever a need or desire to determine a specific patient's radiation dose delivered in a mammography examination, it can be determined in several ways. The three main methods are called the Dance method (Dance et al. 2009), the Wu method (Wu et al. 1994), and the Boone method (Boone 2002).

The following equation is a generalized version of the three methods and can be used to calculate the mean glandular dose for a particular radiation exposure.

$$D_g = D_{gN} \times K$$

where
D_g is the absorbed dose in milligray (mGy);
K is the incident air kerma, to the skin surface, in mGy;
D_{gN} is determined by experimental procedures and depends on:
radiation quality – kVp and HVL
target/filter material
breast thickness
Tissue composition: dense, fatty, or average and if an implant is present.

Most modern digital mammography units calculate an approximation of the mean glandular dose for each image projection and write this information into the DICOM image file header. Different manufacturers select different calculation methods, primarily based on matching the target/filter material composition used by the authors in determining their method.

In Figure 3.13, some DICOM header information is shown. From that image, some relevant data for the mean glandular dose calculation are:

- kVp: 28
- anode material: tungsten
- filter material: rhodium
- compressed BT: 42 mm
- HVL: 0.526 mm of Al
- Entrance dose: 2.86 mGy
- Implant: No

The calculated mean glandular dose, also stored in the DICOM header, was 0.0101 mGy.

Some researchers (Suleiman et al. 2017) studied the accuracy of the calculated mean glandular dose in the image file header. In all mammography units, typically there was an over or under-calculation of the dose. They also concluded that the calculated mean glandular dose could be used as an estimator and was a good audit method between mammography units of the same make and model.

Typical Doses

Mammographers/mammography technologists and radiologists should have enough knowledge of radiation physics and effects to discuss the possible risks associated with the diagnostic exposures with their patients. A few radiation facts should be known to all radiation workers and they are:

- The average effective dose from background radiation varies significantly between locations. Some examples of background (averaged for that country) are
    - United States, approximately 3.0 mSv (300 mrem) per year.
    - United Kingdom, approximately 2.0 mSv (200 mrem) per year.
    - Canada, approximately 1.8 mSv (180 mrem) per year.
    - Australia, approximately 1.7 mSv (170 mrem) per year.
    - The world, approximately 2.4 mSv (240 mrem) per year and the dose can be as high as 12.5 mSv on the Kerala Coast in India
- Sources of background radiation are:
    - Air, mainly radon gas. Colder climate areas tend to have higher doses from radon gas as warmer climate areas tend to have more open windows and doors in houses/apartments.

- Food and water. For example, carbon (C) is one of the most abundant elements in human bodies and ^{14}C is a radioisotope. Food, especially bananas, contain potassium (K) and ^{40}K is a radioisotope.
- Ground, called terrestrial radiation. For example, there are small amounts of uranium and thorium in most soils.
- Cosmic radiation from space. The amount depends on the height above sea level and higher levels of exposure occur during plane flights.
- Another source of ionizing radiation exposure is from man-made sources. The *population dose*, the average dose to a population, for example, in a country, is made of the background radiation and an average of the doses from medical and other man-made sources.
- Annual dose limit exists for occupational workers, including mammographers/mammography technologists, and for members of the public. Most countries have adopted the dose limits from the International Atomic Energy Agency (IAEA) 2014 standard, the Radiation Protection and Safety of Radiation Sources: International Basic Safety Standards, General Safety Requirements Part 3. The limits are
  - Occupational exposure of workers, an effective dose of 20 mSv per year averaged over five consecutive years and 50 mSv in any single year.
  - Members of the public, an effective dose of 1 mSv in a year.
  - Both exclude radiation doses from background radiation and medical examinations.
- The IAEA General Safety Requirements Part 3 states that there are three general principles of radiation protection. These are
  - Justification: All medical radiation exposure needs to be justified. This should be based on a risk versus benefit basis and typically done by the referring

physician. Screening mammography programs are an example of where a person (the client) can self-refer without input from a physician. Here the justification is undertaken at a government or similar level to determine the risk versus benefit, for both the individual and the population.

- Optimization: In mammography, this is the role of the mammographer/mammography technologist. Education, training, and ongoing training constitute a fundamental part of the knowledge and skills needed for optimization. This is also known by the acronym, ALARA, which is As Low As Reasonably Achievable, taking into account social and economic factors.
- Dose limits: For occupational and public exposure, the limits are set and details are provided above. For medical examinations or treatment, there are no limits. However, several approaches can be used. They are
  - Dose reference levels (DRLs): DRLs are a benchmark for radiology departments/practices to review their radiologic examination dose levels against. DRLs are typically set at the 75th percentile of the doses reported for the same examination/projection with a minimum sample size of 50 examinations. As an example, the European DRL is 2 mGy for a compressed breast thickness of 45 mm.
  - A national dose level: In the United States, the Food and Drug Administration (FDA) in their Mammography Quality Standard Act (MQSA) has set a dose limit of 3 mGy (300 mrad) per projection. This is a level that is rarely exceeded for digital mammography, digital breast tomosynthesis, and photon counting mammography.

■ Typical breast imaging doses reported in a range of literature are:

  ■ Full-field digital mammography (FFDM): the dose differs significantly depending on breast thickness and ranges from 0.5 to over 5.0 mGy per projection. A commonly quoted dose range, from the IAEA, for digital mammography examinations involving two views of each breast is that such a breast imaging examination has a total dose to the glandular tissue (D_g) of between 3 and 5 mGy.

  ■ Digital breast tomosynthesis (DBT): the dose of DBT is higher than FFDM for a single FFDM view and a single DBT examination. This is typically a 30–40% increase. However, clinically only one DBT examination/projection of each breast may be needed, whereas for FFDM, two views of each breast are always undertaken. In this case, the total breast dose of DBT will be slightly lower than a FFDM examination. Similar to FFDM, DBT dose significantly differs depending on breast thickness. Also, clinically, the use of DBT can have advantages over FFDM.

  ■ Photon-counting mammography (PCM): the dose of PCM is approximately one-half to one-third of the dose of FFDM per projection.

Putting Radiation Dose in Perspective

Life is full of risks. Every day people voluntarily submit themselves to risks that are much greater than the risks associated with diagnostic-level radiation doses (e.g. driving a car, smoking cigarettes, and being overweight). Knowledge about the health risks of radiation can help put the risks in perspective.

Health Risks of Radiation

- ■ High doses of radiation are known to be detrimental to health. However, radiation doses from most medical imaging examinations are very low and the risks from high radiation doses such as death, radiation burns, and cataracts of the eye are extremely low, and essentially nonexistent from breast imaging.
- ■ A typical effective dose for a mammogram of both breasts is 0.36 mSv (from a typical absorbed dose of 3 mGy – see above), and depending on location, is equivalent to approximately six weeks of background radiation.
- ■ Published risks for diagnostic doses are hypothetical and are calculated based on the known effects of large radiation exposures using the most conservative (linear; no threshold) hypothesis for extrapolation.
- ■ A typical analysis of the hypothetical risk of inducing fatal cancer from undergoing mammography can be as follows:
- ■ A conservative risk of inducing a fatal cancer with radiation is taken to be 4×10^{-4} per 10 mSv (1 rem), which means that 1 out of 2,500 persons receiving 10 mSv of effective dose (whole-body) may die from a cancer that was caused by the radiation. Note, the latency period or time of cancer induction is approximately 7 years for leukemia and 10 years for solid cancers.
- ■ Table 5.2 shows the estimates of breast cancer incidence and mortality for women receiving a dose of 10 mGy to both breasts.
- ■ Example of risk in screening mammography:
    - ■ A typical effective dose from screening mammography examination, shown above, is 0.36 mSv (36 mrem). This radiation level produces a risk of fatal cancer induction for screening mammography of approximately $0.36 \text{ mSv} \times (4 \times 10^{-4}$ per $10 \text{ mSv}) = 14 \times 10^{-6}$ (14 per million).

Table 5.2 US National Academy of Sciences Biologic Effects of Ionizing Radiation (BEIR) VII Report. Estimates of Breast Cancer Incidence and Mortality in Females by Age at Exposure. Risks Are Stated in the Number of Radiation-Caused Cancer Cases or Deaths per Million Women Exposed to 10 mGy to Both Breasts

Age, in Years, at Exposure	Risk of Cancer Incident/Million	Risk of Cancer Mortality/Million
15	553	130
20	429	101
30	253	61
40	141	35
50	70	19
60	31	9
70	12	5
80	4	2

Source: Adapted from Hendrick (2020)

- If an individual has screening mammography every year for 40 years, then the risk of inducing a fatal cancer becomes approximately $14 \times 10^{-6} \times 40$ or approximately 5.76×10^{-4} ($\approx$ 6 per 10,000).

Shielding During Mammography Examination

- Thyroid shielding: The thyroid is relatively close to the breasts during a mammogram and does receive a very low amount of backscatter during the examination. The risk of developing thyroid cancer from multiple mammograms over many years is very low. Thyroid shields are sometimes used, however, there is a risk of repeating the examination due to the shielding blocking some anatomy. Thyroid shielding should be considered for mammograms of young women.

■ Pregnancy: It is generally accepted that the dose to a fetus during a mammographic examination is very low, and well below the dose levels that will or can cause fetal harm or development issues. However, it is recommended that:

■ diagnostic mammography is undertaken during pregnancy only after greater thought and consideration of the radiation protection principles of justification, and not undertaken in screening mammography.

■ lead apron shielding should be worn by the patient.

Putting It All Together

Screening mammography of an individual for 40 years has the potential to induce a fatal cancer in approximately 6 out of 10,000 individuals. However, in these same 10,000 women, by age 80, there may be, for example, 1,000 cases of breast cancer. If only half of the cancers can be detected and treated (including any that may have been induced), about 500 cancer deaths may be prevented by screening mammography.

This simplistic presentation involves some assumptions and uncertainties, but the following point should be understood clearly: *the risks associated with good screening mammography, although not zero, are low and are much less than the risks of undetected cancer.*

Several steps can be taken to decrease the radiation dose delivered to the population by mammography, the most obvious being to quit mammography. However, currently, in developed countries around the world, there is a consensus that the benefits of annual screening mammography, typically beginning at age 40, clearly outweigh the risks. The current priority for screening mammography is early and accurate detection of breast cancer.

Other steps have been and are being taken to reduce the dose in all mammography examinations. The first step was/is the transition from film/screen mammography to digital mammography. Other dose reduction methods such as photon counting mammography, grid need and design, and dose reduction research are being evaluated, however, image quality and diagnostic efficacy cannot be compromised.

Bibliography

Ali, R. M. K., England, A., Tootell, A. K. and Hogg, P. (2020). "Radiation dose from digital breast tomosynthesis screening – a comparison with full field digital mammography." *Journal of Medical Imaging and Radiation Sciences* 51(4): 599–603.

Asbeutah, A. M., AlMajran, A. A., Brindhaban, A. and Asbeutah, S. A. (2020). "Comparison of radiation doses between diagnostic full-field digital mammography (FFDM) and digital breast tomosynthesis (DBT): a clinical study." *Journal of Medical Radiation Sciences* 67(3): 185–192.

Boone, J. M. (2002). "Normalized glandular dose (DgN) coefficients for arbitrary X-ray spectra in mammography: computer-fit values of Monte Carlo derived data." *Medical Physics* 29(5): 869–875.

Bor, D., Tukel, S., Olgar, T., Toklu, T., Aydın, E. and Akyol, O. (2008). "Investigation of mean glandular dose versus compressed breast thickness relationship for mammography." *Radiation Protection Dosimetry* 129(1–3): 160–164.

Dance, D. and Young, K. (2014). "Estimation of mean glandular dose for contrast enhanced digital mammography: factors for use with the UK, European and IAEA breast dosimetry protocols." *Physics in Medicine & Biology* 59(9): 2127.

Dance, D. R., Young, K. C. and van Engen, R. E. (2009). "Further factors for the estimation of mean glandular dose using the United Kingdom, European and IAEA breast dosimetry protocols." *Physics in Medicine and Biology* 54(14): 4361–4372.

Dance, D. R., Young, K. C. and van Engen, R. E. (2011). "Estimation of mean glandular dose for breast tomosynthesis: factors for use with the UK, European and IAEA breast dosimetry protocols." *Physics in Medicine and Biology* 56(2): 453–471.

Gennaro, G., Bernardi, D. and Houssami, N. (2018). "Radiation dose with digital breast tomosynthesis compared to digital mammography: per-view analysis." *European Radiology* 28(2): 573–581.

Hendrick, R. E. (2020). "Radiation doses and risks in breast screening." *Journal of Breast Imaging* 2(3): 188–200.

ICRP Publication 103 (2007). International Commission on Radiological Protection.

International Atomic Energy Agency (2014). *Radiation Protection and Safety of Radiation Sources: International Basic Safety Standards, General Safety Requirements Part 3*. Vienna, International Atomic Energy Agency.

Kieturakis, A. J., Wahab, R. A., Vijapura, C. and Mahoney, M. C. (2021). "Current recommendations for breast imaging of the pregnant and lactating patient." *American Journal of Roentgenology* 216(6): 1462–1475.

Liu, Q., Suleiman, M. E., McEntee, M. F. and Soh, B. P. (2022). "Diagnostic reference levels in digital mammography: a systematic review." *Journal of Radiological Protection* 42(1): 11503.

Mettler, F. A. Jr., Huda, W., Yoshizumi, T. T. and Mahesh, M. (2008). "Effective doses in radiology and diagnostic nuclear medicine: a catalog." *Radiology* 248(1): 254–263.

Nosratieh, A., Hernandez, A., Shen, S. Z., Yaffe, M. J., Seibert, J. A. and Boone, J. M. (2015). "Mean glandular dose coefficients (DgN) for x-ray spectra used in contemporary breast imaging systems." *Physics in Medicine & Biology* 60(18): 7179.

Olgar, T., Kahn, T. and Gosch, D. (2012). Average glandular dose in digital mammography and breast tomosynthesis. *RöFo-Fortschritte auf dem Gebiet der Röntgenstrahlen und der bildgebenden Verfahren*. © Georg Thieme Verlag KG.

Pyka, M., Eschle, P., Sommer, C., Weyland, M. S., Kubik, R. and Scheidegger, S. (2018). "Effect of thyroid shielding during mammography: measurements on phantom and patient as well as estimation with Monte Carlo simulation." *European Radiology Experimental* 2: 14.

Seeram, E. and Brennan, P. (2016). *Radiation Protection in Diagnostic X-Ray Imaging*. Burlington, MA, Jones & Bartlett Learning.

Suleiman, M., Brennan, P. and McEntee, M. (2017). "Mean glandular dose in digital mammography: a dose calculation method comparison." *Journal of Medical Imaging* 4(1): 013502.

Weigel, S., Berkemeyer, S., Girnus, R., Sommer, A., Lenzen, H. and Heindel, W. (2014). "Digital mammography screening with photon-counting technique: can a high diagnostic performance be realized at low mean glandular dose?" *Radiology* 271(2): 345–355.

Wu, X., Gingold, E. L., Barnes, G. T. and Tucker, D. M. (1994). "Normalized average glandular dose in molybdenum target-rhodium filter and rhodium target-rhodium filter mammography." *Radiology* 193(1): 83–89.

6 Mammographic Image Quality

Chapter at a Glance

- Introduction
- Clinical Image Quality Requirements
- Image Quality in Mammography
- Spatial Resolution
- Image Contrast
- Noise
- Relationships Among Spatial Resolution, Image Contrast, and Noise
- Artifacts
- Quality Control and Quality Assurance
- Bibliography

Introduction

This chapter is not about the assessment of clinical mammography image quality that all mammographers/mammography technologists should undertake, for example, using the PGMI (Perfect, Good, Moderate, Inadequate) method for evaluation

Digital Mammography: Physics and Instrumentation, Second Edition.
Rob Davidson.
© 2026 John Wiley & Sons Ltd. Published 2026 by John Wiley & Sons Ltd.

of clinical image quality. The foci of such a method are on patient/client positioning, adequate compression, and technical appearance such as correct exposure factors, absence of movement, and artifacts of the mammogram.

The focus here is on technical factors inherent in the imaging system that are needed to have high-quality mammographic images.

Clinical Image Quality Requirements

What do radiologists see in the image that allows them to make a diagnosis of breast pathology such as breast cancers, benign tumors, and cysts? The following section is not meant to be a lesson on mammographic interpretation; rather, it provides a few of the important mammographic image features of pathologies and as such explains the high levels of quality that are needed in mammographic examinations.

High-Density Masses

A mass that has high density, compared with adipose tissue, can be benign or malignant. A high tissue density results from greater attenuation of the X-ray photons and will appear brighter in the image than adipose and other tissues. The features of the mass, in particular, its shape and the characteristics of its margin provide clues that allow differentiation of benign and malignant masses.

- A benign mass will typically present the following characteristics:
  - round or oval shape
  - smooth, well-demarcated, and completely visualized margin
  - sharply defined border sometimes surrounded by a halo
- The most common benign breast masses are fibroadenomas and cysts.

- Indications suggesting malignancy include the following:
    - irregular or lobulated shape or both
    - indistinct, fuzzy, or non-visualized margin
    - indentations in the margin (occasionally referred to as the tent sign).
    - spiculations, spokes, or tentacle-like radiations extending from the mass.

The spiculations associated with breast cancer are likely a result of an enzyme imbalance caused by cancer that travels out along fibrous tissue planes to produce the classic spoked or spiked appearance.

Microcalcifications

Approximately 50% of the cancers detected with mammography produce calcifications. This number of cancer cases is important because the cancers detected by micro-calcifications are usually less advanced. As with masses, breast calcifications can be either benign or malignant. The characteristics of benign calcifications are similar to the characteristics of benign masses, including the following:

- round, smooth shape
- well-defined
- occasionally a lucent center

Common causes of benign calcifications are:

- mastitis
- Milk of calcium: Milk of calcium is dissolved calcium in the fluid within the acini at the terminus of the milk ducts and can be diagnosed by comparing the cranio-caudal (CC) view with the lateral-oblique view. In the CC view, the calcifications will be round and in the lateral view, they will have a teacup appearance.

Calcifications caused by cancer are a result of the death of cells lining the terminal ducts. The dying cells spew their contents, including calcium, into the duct. The shape and distribution of calcifications can provide important indicators of their origin:

- linear patterns of calcification and linear branching patterns of calcification can be indicative of cancer.
    - When the linear or branching patterns are solid, referred to as rodlike, the calcification could be a result of calcified ducts caused by secretory disease, another benign condition.
    - When the linear or branched linear structures resemble a dotted line, the probability of cancer increases.
- the shape of malignant calcifications in a mammogram has been described as crushed stone or broken needle tip.
- another term often used to describe a cluster of malignant calcifications is pleomorphic, designating a variety of sizes and shapes.

Architectural Distortion

Skin dimpling or nipple retraction can be described as advanced architectural distortion. However, long before these features are visible externally, the normal parenchymal architecture will likely be disturbed by the disease process. Mammographers/mammography technologists who have performed a great deal of mammography have learned to recognize the typical parenchymal patterns of normal breast tissue. Features that do not follow the expected pattern may provide important clues that will aid in finding a subtle cancer. For example:

- a concave instead of convex trajectory
- straight or linear structure, appearing stretched
- a radiating pattern resembling spokes in a wheel

Image Quality in Mammography

Image quality has four main areas, three of which are strongly interrelated, known as the image quality triangle, as shown in Figure 6.1. These three factors of image quality are image contrast, spatial resolution, and noise. One factor alone is no more important than the others and the diagrams try to stress that link between them. The fourth factor, not shown in Figure 6.1, is image artifacts, the presence of which can also reduce image quality.

An example of one image quality factor alone not being more important than the others is that in current full-field digital mammography (FFDM) or 2D mammography, spatial resolution is stated as being between 7 and 10 line-pairs per millimeter (lp/mm). A discussion on lp/mm will be done later. When mammographic images were captured using film/screen methods, the spatial resolution of a good imaging system

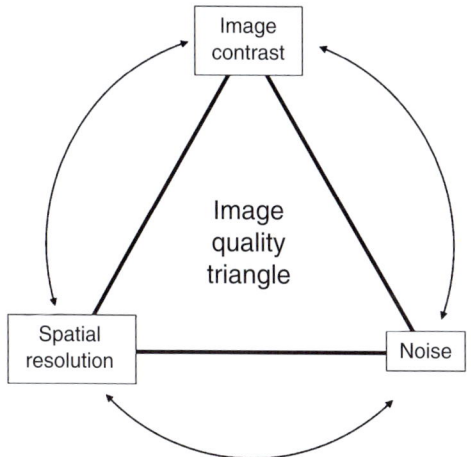

Figure 6.1 The image quality triangle showing three of the main factors of image quality, image contrast, spatial resolution, and noise.

was stated as 20 lp/mm, which is twice or more than FFDM. When moving away from film/screen to FFDM, spatial resolution was reduced yet the diagnostic ability of FFDM did not diminish, and most researchers state diagnostic ability is actually improved. This improved diagnostic ability is primarily due to the improved image contrast and digital image processing (DIP) enhancements, such as noise reduction and edge enhancement of objects, that improve the viewer's ability to visualize small objects.

Spatial Resolution

Spatial resolution refers to the ability of an imaging system to separate small objects that are close together. The most commonly used tool to assess spatial resolution in X-ray imaging is a line-pair phantom, a series of high attenuating strips and low attenuating gaps, known as line-pairs, of various sizes. The smallest set of line-pairs seen in the image without degradation is the measure of the imaging system's spatial resolution.

Spatial resolution is often reported in lp/mm and measured using a line-pair phantom. An example of a line-pair phantom is seen in Figure 6.2, showing lines from 0.5 to 14 lp/mm. Line-pair phantoms will use lead as the attenuating material and air as the gap. An example of converting lp/mm into the size of imaged detail can be seen when using a line-pair phantom and the 10 lp/mm area of the phantom is visualized. Ten line-pairs indicate 10 lines and 10 spaces of equal size. The imaged detail can be equated to the size of a resolved line. Because there are a total of 20 lines and spaces in a millimeter, each line and space are 1/50 mm which is 0.05 mm or 50 μm or microns.

Other measures of spatial resolution that can be used in X-ray imaging, though not discussed here, are the point spread function (PSF), line spread function (LSF), and edge spread function (ESF). These measures are often used by physicists when researching mammography image quality.

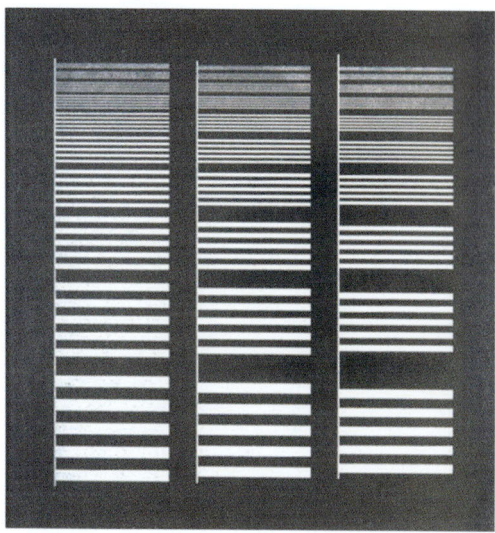

Figure 6.2 A line-pair phantom with line-pair sizes from 0.5 to 14 lp/mm.

The flat panel detector (FPD) thin film transistor (TFT) pixel size in all current mammography units is fixed. The FPD pixel size, or the pixel density, stated as the number of pixels per millimeter, is the limiting spatial resolution of the system. The photon number values are recorded one-for-one into the image matrix and as such no magnification or minification between the FPD and the image occurs and no loss of spatial resolution occurs during conversion to an image.

The image spatial resolution of the image however can be improved above the FPD pixel size. In magnification mode, the size of the object in the image does increase and it is possible to visualize more lp/mm in magnification mode compared to normal mode.

In mammography, the spatial resolution of the system is monitored using specially designed phantoms (more on these later in this chapter). The most common phantoms are those approved by the American College of Radiology (ACR). These phantoms have fiber lines and specs of varying small sizes, and a minimum

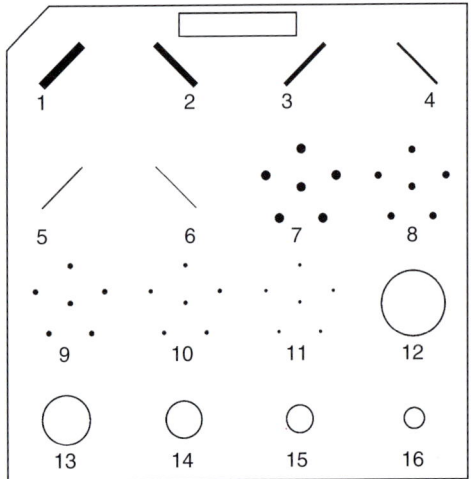

Figure 6.3 A diagram of an ACR-approved phantom, the CIRS Model 015. In the phantom, fiber (objects 1–6) widths are between 0.4 and 1.56 mm, specks (objects 7–11) sizes between 0.16 and 0.54 mm, and objects 12–16 thicknesses between 0.25 and 2.0 mm.

size must be visualized in the image to meet spatial resolution requirements and accreditation standards. Figure 6.3 shows a diagram of the structures of an ACR-approved phantom, the CIRS Model 015.

In digital mammography, two groups of factors affect spatial resolution. These groups are physical factors and image processing factors.

The physical factors are:

- Effective focal spot size, which is affected by the:
  - actual focal spot size
  - anode angle
  - position in the X-ray field along the cathode-anode axis of the field
  - cathode focusing cup bias, used to control blooming of the actual focal spot size

- Geometry and magnification factor:
  - geometric unsharpness, formally known as penumbra, is the blurring seen at the edge of an object in the image where the actual object has a highly defined edge. This is caused by two factors which are
    - the size of the effective focal spot. If the focal spot was infinitely small, that is, a point source, then there would be no geometric unsharpness or blurring of the edges of objects in the image. As all focal spots have a finite size, some geometric unsharpness will occur. The smaller the source-to-image distance (SID), the less the geometric unsharpness.
    - a finite distance between the actual object and the recording device, in this case, the FPD. This distance is the SID. The smaller the SID, the less the geometric unsharpness.
  - magnification = SID ÷ source-to-object distance (SOD). The magnification in standard mode mammography is typically 1.05–1.10; in the magnification mode, the magnification is typically between 1.5 and 2.0.
  - object–image distance (OID) is equal to the SID minus the SOD. A larger OID corresponds to higher magnification.
  - in magnification mode, imaging requires the use of the small focal spot to minimize geometric unsharpness/penumbra.
  - compressing the breast tissues reduces the magnification factor, reduces geometric unsharpness, and improves spatial resolution.
  - breast thickness is a factor in magnification. Thicker breasts and breast features located superior in the breast, that is, closer to the X-ray tube, are imaged with higher magnification than the breast's inferior structures.

- Motion:

  Motion can be a problem in mammography. Motion is visualized as blur which decreases the spatial resolution of the image. The factors that contribute to the probability of motion in a mammogram include:

  - Exposure time: This is affected by the
    - mA that is used. The automatic exposure control (AEC) will terminate the exposure when the required number of photons reaches the FPD. As such using a higher mA will reduce exposure time.
    - focal spot selected. The large focal spot has a higher mA output than the small focal spot.
    - kVp selected. Increasing the kVp increases the radiation output for a given mA. Using the kVp rule, a 15% increase in the kVp approximately doubles the number of photons produced.
      - kVp/target/filter selection. As discussed in Chapter 2, increasing the kVp when the target/filter combination is tungsten (W)/silver (Ag) primarily increases the number of X-ray photons in the beam and only minimally increases the beam's average energy.
    - target/filter combination. Different target/filter combination affects the average energy of the photons in the X-ray beam. A higher average energy will reduce the number of photons being attenuated in the breast, increasing the number reaching the FPD and hence reducing the time needed for the imaging.
    - the maximum power of a generator and output of the X-ray tube; varies from manufacturer to manufacturer.
    - breast thickness and composition; thicker and denser breasts require more exposure

thus a longer exposure time for the same kVp, target/filter combination, and mA setting.
- a compressed breast is a thinner breast and has less attenuation than an uncompressed breast, hence requiring less exposure and can have a shorter exposure time.

The image processing factors. Some examples are:

- Digital magnification or image zoom: Digital magnification can improve the viewer's ability to visualize small objects in the image. This improved visualization is known as an increase in perceived spatial resolution. Digital magnification does not improve physical spatial resolution, as the recorded pixel values are mathematically spread over more display pixels.
- Edge enhancements processes: Again, these do not improve physical spatial resolution but do increase the viewer's ability to visualize small objects in the image.

Image Contrast

Image contrast of a system or contrast resolution refers to the ability of an imaging system to differentiate between large objects. A broad measure of contrast between two objects in an image is

- the pixel value of object A – the pixel value of object B/ pixel value of object A (or the background)

In digital imaging, there needs to be a pixel value difference between objects; otherwise, no matter what image processing is used, the two areas will be displayed with the same level of gray on the monitor.

In mammography, image contrast/contrast resolution of the system is also monitored using ACR-approved phantoms. The same phantom that is used for spatial resolution also has large, a few centimeters in size, objects. The resultant image must be able to differentiate between two similar attenuating objects to meet accreditation standards.

Image contrast is dependent on several factors, and these are the subject contrast, scatter radiation, and image processing and display.

Subject Contrast

Subject contrast is defined for this text to be the attenuation differences in irradiated tissue and is determined by both the energy of the X-ray beam and the tissue characteristics. This has been previously discussed in Chapter 3, and the main points are given below.

- Average or effective X-ray beam energy: The main factors are:
  - kVp
  - voltage ripple factor
  - target material
  - filter material and thickness.

High average X-ray beam energy generally means low subject contrast and vice versa.

- Breast and other tissue composition:
  - A small difference in attenuation characteristics exists between fibroglandular and adipose tissue and between these tissues and pathologies.
  - Breast density.
    There are four breast density classifications as defined by the ACR's Breast Imaging-Reporting and Data System (BI-RADS). They are
    - Fatty: the breasts are almost entirely adipose tissue. Typically, older women have fatty breasts.
    - Scattered fibroglandular: there are scattered areas of fibroglandular density with the adipose tissue.

- Heterogeneously dense: the breasts are approximately an equal mix of fibroglandular and adipose tissues.
- Extremely dense: the breasts are predominantly fibroglandular tissues. Typically, young women have extremely dense breasts.
- The effective atomic numbers and densities have very small differences (also see Chapter 1) and are for:
  - Adipose tissues – approx. 6.0 and 0.90 g/cm^3
  - Fibroglandular tumor tissues – approx. 7.0 and 0.96 g/cm^3
  - Tumor tissues – approx. 7.4 and 1.07 g/cm^3
- Calcium: Calcium has higher attenuation characteristics than glandular and adipose tissues due to its atomic number of 20. However, calcifications are small, and therefore other factors such as spatial resolution and image noise can degrade their visibility in the image.

Scattered Radiation

Scattered radiation and control methods have been discussed in Chapter 3. Scattered radiation results from the interaction of the X-ray photons with the atoms in the breast tissue. It is distributed close to evenly across the anatomy in the image (there is some non-uniformity) and when reaching the FPD adds to the pixel value.

Scattered radiation is detrimental to image quality primarily by reducing image contrast. An example to show the reduction of image contrast is:

Without any scatter:

Pixel 1 value = 100,
Pixel 2 value = 120.
Contrast (the percentage difference them) =
(120 − 100) ÷ 100 (Pixel 1 value) = 20%

Scatter adds a value of 20 to all pixels.
With scatter:

> Pixel 1 value = 120,
> Pixel 2 value = 140.
> Contrast = (140 − 120) ÷ 120 (Pixel 1 value) = 16.7%.

A list of the main scatter control means is:

- X-ray beam energy:
  The production of scattered radiation is slightly greater for higher X-ray beam energies but is not a major factor in mammography.
- Volume of tissue irradiated:
  The larger the quantity of tissue that is irradiated by X-rays, the more scattered radiation is produced. The volume of tissue irradiated depends on three factors:
    - Breast thickness: Breast compression results in less scatter being produced compared to an uncompressed breast. The X-ray beam has a shorter path length/distance to travel in the breast; hence, there is less probability of scattering.
    - Radiation field size: The smaller the volume of tissue, the less scatter. Spot collimation results in less scattered radiation being produced (and has increased compression/reduced breast thickness compared to standard mammography compression).
- Breast composition:
  There is a small difference between fibroglandular and adipose tissue scatter characteristics; however, this is only a small contributing factor. It is also something that is not under the control of the mammographer undertaking the mammographic examination.
- Grids:
  Use of a grid will reduce scatter radiation reaching the FPD.

- Air Gap:
  Use of an air gap will reduce scatter radiation reaching the FPD.
- Digital image processing techniques:
  Techniques of scatter correction or removal from the image have been tried and are starting to be used. The process is essentially to model scatter distribution for different breast sizes, thickness, densities, and X-ray factors of kVp and anode/filter combinations. The model of the scatter is then subtracted from the breast image that has scatter radiation in the image.

Image Processing and Display Factors

The main factors are:

- Detector noise:
  While detector noise is generally not high, and not as high as the scatter radiation contribution even when a grid is used, and as such the reduction of image contrast from detector noise is small.
- Pre-processing/transformation process:
  Once the FPD has recorded the pixel values, pre-processing or the transformation process occurs to convert the raw pixel values to image values. See Chapter 3 for more details on this process. In this process, there can be errors in determining the appropriate transformation look-up table (LUT) for that breast anatomy. Given breast anatomical shape is more consistent between patients and is placed consistently on the FPD than in other anatomical areas in general radiography, the transformation process in mammography is more robust than in general radiography.

- Displayed image contrast:
  Displayed image contrast can be altered by the use of window width (WW) functions controlled by the viewer. As discussed in Chapter 3, which has more details on this, the look-up-tables (LUT) used in mammography are sigmoid shaped.

Noise

Noise is a variation in pixel values in areas of the image where the signal does not vary. In X-ray imaging and mammography, the signal is the transmitted primary X-ray photons reaching and being recorded by the FPD. A variation of pixel values will be visualized as variations of shades of gray or speckled appearances in a uniform area of the displayed image.

Noise is measured as a ratio of the signal and the noise. This is the signal-to-noise ratio (SNR). This is not an easy measurement to make and, if needed, is measured by physicists. An alternate measure of image quality and noise is the signal difference-to-noise ratio (SDNR).

Noise however does degrade both spatial resolution and image contrast. An ACR-approved phantom that is used for evaluating spatial resolution and image contrast can have these small and large objects degraded by noise, so their visibility in the image is reduced.

Noise also has both external and internal image contributors. The external contributors are:

- Scatter radiation:
  Scatter radiation when reaching the FPD and adding to the pixel value is an unwanted value. As such, it is noise. Scatter production is also a random event and while generally evenly spread across the FPD, there are variations in scatter intensities between pixels.

Scatter reduction methods, discussed above and in Chapter 3, are needed.

- Variations in primary radiation:

An assumption in X-ray imaging and mammography is that the unattenuated X-ray beam is uniform across the entire X-ray field when reaching the FPD. It is recognized that there is a variation in the X-ray beam's intensity from the anode heel effect (discussed in Chapter 2) in the anode–cathode direction of the field. There are always variations in the unattenuated X-ray beam's intensity not related to the anode heel effect and this is known as Poisson noise.

In the early days of film/screen radiography, Poisson noise was also called mottle. Its appearance is a so-called salt-and-pepper appearance where there are small lighter and darker areas in a uniform area of the image. This Poisson noise/salt-and-pepper appearance becomes more obvious in the image when the number of primary photons is low. Many factors cause low photon numbers, the prime being a low tube current (mA), especially when imaging a larger object. The low number of primary photons (low signal) will result in a low SNR/SDNR given the same level of noise present in the image. The use of appropriate exposure settings for each individual patient will minimize Poisson noise/mottle.

- Detector and electronic noise:

Noise from the detectors and the system's electronics will always be present. The materials chosen for the detectors are optimized to reduce this noise. The detective quantum efficiency (DQE) of the detector, discussed in Chapter 3, is an indirect measure of the noise resulting from the detectors themselves. Similar to the above, the use of appropriate exposure settings and having an appropriate level of signal (primary radiation) minimize any appearance of this noise.

The internal image contributors are mainly from DIP processes. These are:

- Edge enhancement:
  The use of unsharp masks increases noise. Edge enhancement processes are designed to improve the visualization of small objects in the image. Noise, especially salt-and-pepper noise, are small areas in the image and the unsharp mask will enhance the pixel values in the noise and make the noise more obvious to a viewer of the image. It is important for viewers who edge enhance the image to do this to an appropriate level so as to not make noise in the image more apparent.

  Similarly, multiscale processing can enhance noise in the image.
- Digital zoom:
  Enlarging areas of the image to better view small objects in the image also enlarges and can make noise more apparent in the image.

Relationships Among Spatial Resolution, Image Contrast, and Noise

Figure 6.1 shows the image quality triangle and arrows are seen in both directions between the factors of spatial resolution, image contrast, and noise. Each of these factors is affected by changes in the other factors, usually a degradation of one will degrade the other.

Image Contrast and Noise

Where there is high contrast and a high difference in pixel values between two objects in an image, the small variations of pixel values (grays in the image) will not significantly affect the observer's ability to visualize and differentiate between the two objects.

However, where there is low contrast between two objects in an image, the small variations of the pixel values caused by the noise can make these two objects appear to have the same densities or grays in the image and it is then hard to differentiate between the two objects.

A measure of this relationship between image contrast and noise is the contrast-to-noise ratio (CNR). Optimizing exposure techniques will optimize the images' CNR. CNR is a more useful measure of image quality than SNR and it is easier to measure. As such, it is often the measure of choice used by researchers in evaluating X-ray and mammographic image quality.

Noise in mammography can be monitored. If the large objects are not differentiated in images of ACR-approved phantoms, then noise is a likely cause, and as such noise can evaluated using the ACR-approved phantoms.

Spatial Resolution and Image Contrast

As spatial resolution increases, image contrast decreases. All edges of objects in an image have some level of blur. For a given amount of edge blur on all objects, as the object becomes smaller, the edges of the object start to overlap each other and the overall pixel value in what was at the center of the object is reduced. Similarly, as small objects get closer together, their edges blur together and reduce the objects' pixel value. In both cases, a lower object value compared to the background means the contrast between these two is reduced. An example of this is shown in Figure 6.4. In this figure, an image of line-pair phantom (top) is evaluated using a transect histogram (the pixel values versus distance along the yellow line). On the left side of the line-pair phantom, the objects (line-pairs) are larger and on the right side, they are smaller and closer together. On the right of the histogram, the difference between the objects' pixel values and the background (the contrast between these two) is seen. On the right side of the histogram, pixel value difference/contrast is reduced.

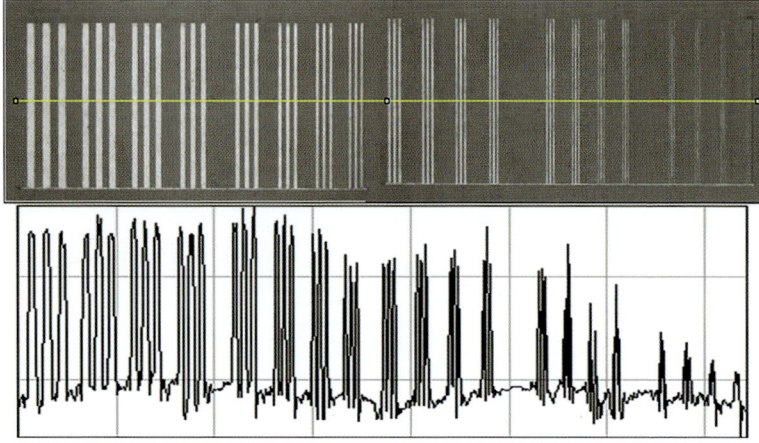

Figure 6.4 A line-pair phantom (top) and corresponding transect histogram of the phantom (bottom).

A means of measuring the relationship between spatial resolution and image contrast is to use a process called modulation transfer function (MTF). Formally, MTF is a measure of the recorded signal (pixel values) divided by the input signal (X-ray photon intensity values) measured over a range of object sizes (spatial frequencies) in lp/mm. As seen above, a decrease in signal intensities versus the background is a reduction of contrast. An example of an MTF plot can be seen in Figure 6.5. The X-axis is the object size (lp/mm) and the Y-axis is the MTF. An MTF value of 1.0 (or 100%) means a perfect transfer of the input signal to pixel values, while less than 1.0 is an imperfect transfer. As objects become smaller (higher lp/mm), the MTF becomes less.

Another means of evaluating this relationship is to take images of a contrast-detail phantom. An example is seen in Figure 6.6. This is the Artinis CDMAM 3.4 phantom and can be used with image analysis software. In this mammography phantom, there is an array of small gold objects of differing sizes

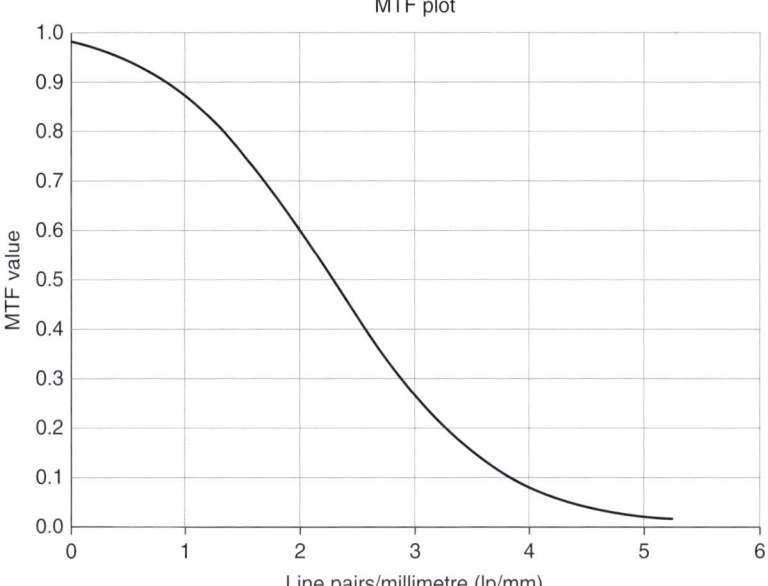

Figure 6.5 A modulation transfer function (MTF) plot of the MTF versus object size in line- pairs/millimeter (lp/mm).

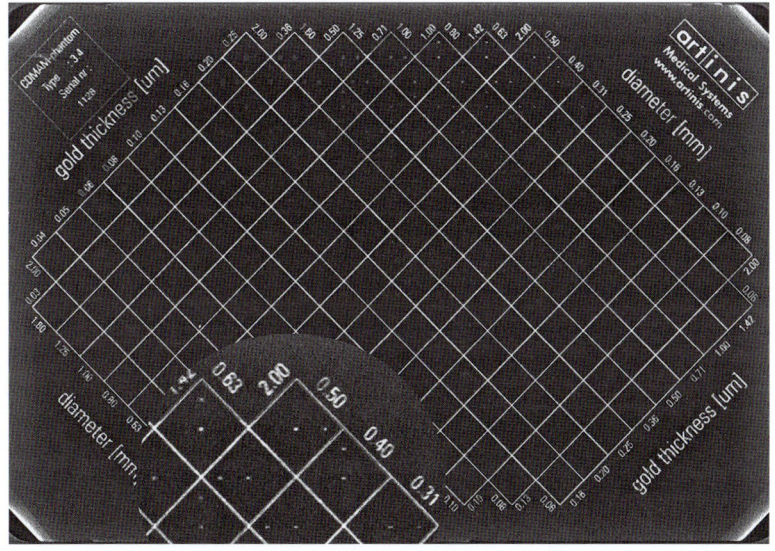

Figure 6.6 Image of a contrast-detail phantom, the Artinis CDMAM 3.4 phantom, with the inset (bottom) showing an enlargement of gold objects of 0.5 mm diameter and 2.0 mm thick.

ranging from 0.06 to 2.0 mm and a thickness of 0.06–2.0 mm. By evaluating the resultant images under various mammographic settings, image quality aspects of spatial resolution and image contrast are reviewed and monitored.

Spatial Resolution and Noise

Noise can both decrease image contrast and cause the edges of objects to appear blurred. Similar to the discussion in the spatial resolution and image contrast section, reduced contrast and blurred edges reduce the spatial resolution. This relationship can be measured and plotted on a Weiner spectrum. A Weiner spectrum essentially plots a value of the noise at different spatial frequencies or object sizes.

Image Quality in Digital Breast Tomosynthesis

Digital breast tomosynthesis (DBT) or 3D mammography, as discussed in Chapter 4, creates images of a thin slice of the breast anatomy at differing heights above the breast support platform. The images are a representation of a thin 3D section of breast thickness. This dimension is the Z-direction/dimension and the image quality in this third dimension, as well as the image quality in the other two dimensions needs to be evaluated and monitored.

An object in the image from this thin slice of the breast needs to have a high spatial resolution, high image contrast, and low noise, and importantly for DBT imaging, it needs to represent the Z or height dimension of the object.

Some existing mammography phantoms can be used to evaluate DBT spatial resolution, image contrast and noise, and the Z-dimension image quality. There are also dedicated phantoms focusing on Z-dimension resolution and image contrast.

Artifacts

Artifacts in medical imaging refer to something seen in an image that is not present in the object being imaged. Artifacts may obscure parts of anatomy/pathology or distort and degrade the image. There are several categories of artifacts. These are:

- Patient-related artifacts:
  These are artifacts that are related to the image of the patient. Some artifacts within this category are:
  - patient movement or motion,
  - clothing,
  - some antiperspirant, talcum powder, skin creams,
  - skinfolds, skin lesions, or other body parts,
  - internal medical devices such as a pacemaker or a port for a central line.
- Equipment-based artifacts:
  These are artifacts not related to the detector, but to the rest of the mammography instrumentation. Some artifacts within this category are:
  - gridlines visible in the image
  - dirt or dust on the compression paddle
  - edges of the compression paddle seen in the image
  - DBT-related artifacts such as streaking appearance of objects
- Detector-based artifacts: Some areas within this category are:
  - Image nonuniformities:
    A flat field image will not be uniformly black and have areas of different greys.
  - Dead pixels/dead or unread lines:
    Will be seen as black spots or lines in the image
  - Ghosting:
    Amorphous selenium (a-Se) detectors can have ghosting problems when cold.

■ Blooming:
Also related to a-Se detectors. This occurs when there is early discharge of a single detector element and a white spot and black halo appearance will be seen.

■ Post-acquisition artifacts: Some areas within this category are:

■ Processing artifacts are artifacts caused by the digital image processing (DIP) algorithm. An example, discussed in Chapter 3, is if the pre-processing or transformation algorithm does not correctly identify the anatomy in the raw histogram, the converted image will not correctly be displayed.

Storage artifacts are artifacts caused when the picture archiving and communication system (PACS) system does not properly display the image. It incorrectly uses information stored within the header for display.

Quality Control and Quality Assurance

Quality control (QC) and quality assurance (QA) are terms that describe a program for improving and maintaining quality. In radiology, definitions taken from Report 99 of the National Council on Radiation Protection and Measurements are:

■ Quality control is a series of distinct technical procedures that ensure the production of a satisfactory product. It aims to provide quality that is not only satisfactory and diagnostic but also dependable and economic.

■ Quality assurance is an all-encompassing program, including quality control, that extends to administrative, educational, and preventative maintenance methods and includes a continuing evaluation of the adequacy and effectiveness of the overall imaging program, to initiate corrective measures when necessary.

QA and QC can help achieve the desired goal of producing consistently high-quality images with the minimal radiation dose necessary to achieve the desired image quality. In nearly every case, the radiation dose can easily be reduced for any given radiologic examination at the expense of reduced image quality. However, patients are irradiated because of the potentially significant benefits to them provided by the examination. Mammographers/mammography technologists should always strive to achieve a maximal image-quality-to-dose ratio (high image quality or low radiation dose). This principle of using the lowest dose consistent with the requirements of the diagnostic examination is often expressed using the acronym ALARA, which means *As Low As Reasonably Achievable* taking into account social and economic factors, and is the radiation protection principle of optimization.

The potential benefits of QC–QA are well-known. However, there are also costs associated with the performance of QC–QA that include time, equipment, and frustration, to mention a few. Some questions that need to be answered are:

■ What technical factors should be tested?
■ How often should these factors be tested?

To answer these questions, two additional questions should be asked:

■ How does this technical factor affect image quality?
■ How likely is image quality to change?

All mammography QC–QA programs and tests must comply with their country's regulations or codes. For example, in the United States, the US Food and Drug Administration (FDA) has established the Mammography Quality Standards Act (MQSA). QC–QA programs in the United States must meet these standards. Some other similar standards or codes are:

- Europe: European Guidelines for Quality Assurance in Breast Cancer Screening and Diagnosis.
- Canada: Canadian Mammography Quality Guidelines.
- Australia/New Zealand: Digital Mammography Quality Assurance Program.

Some recommended annual tests are

- mammography unit assembly evaluation including compression
- generator performance
- focal spot size
- collimation and alignment assessment
- AEC performance
- exposure time
- beam quality or half-value layer
- image quality evaluation including
    - system resolution/MTF
    - ghost image evaluation
    - system linearity and noise analysis image
    - uniformity and artifact evaluation
- mean glandular dose
- monitor luminance and viewing conditions

Personnel Knowledge and Experience/Accreditation

Similar to meeting equipment standards, personnel involved in mammography examinations must meet their country's requirements for mammography knowledge and experience.

Depending on the country, personnel accreditation may then follow. The personnel involved are:

1. Mammographers/mammography radiologic technologists:

- Initial qualifications:
    - be licensed or registered to practice medical imaging/diagnostic radiography in their country/ state as a Radiologic Technologist/Diagnostic Radiographer.
    - be certified/accredited by the country's approved specialty/registry board and
        - have undertaken and completed education in mammography, for example, undertake an approved program of study
        - meet minimum training requirements in mammography, for example, performance of at least 25 exams under qualified direct supervision
- Continuing experience and education:
    - have undertaken minimum mammographic examination requirements in a given timeframe, for example, perform at least 200 exams per two years period following initial qualification
    - have met minimum continuing education (CE)/continuing professional development (CPD) requirements, for example, eight hours of CE/CPD

2. Mammography radiologists/Interpreting physicians:

- Initial qualifications:
    - be licensed or registered to practice medicine in their country/state.
    - be certified/accredited by the country's approved specialty/registry board and
        - meet minimum formal training requirements in mammogram interpretation, for example, three months

- have education in mammography, for example, ≥ 60 hours
- have read and met minimum mammographic examination requirements in a given timeframe, for example, ≥ 240 in the previous six months
- Continuing experience and education:
    - have read and met minimum mammographic examination requirements in a given timeframe, for example, have read ≥ 960 mammographic exams in any two-year period
    - have met minimum continuing education requirements, for example, have 15 credits in any three-year period

3. Medical physicists:

- Initial qualifications:
    - be educated with a bachelor's degree and/or have post-graduate qualifications in medical physics that have a focus on radiology.
    - be certified/accredited by their country's medical physics organization in mammography. Examples of such organizations are
        - American Association of Physicists in Medicine
        - European Federation of Organizations for Medical Physics
        - UK's Institute of Physics and Engineering in Medicine
        - Canadian Organization of Medical Physicists
        - Australia/New Zealand–Australasian College of Physical Scientists and Engineers in Medicine
    - be licensed for the use of ionizing radiation

- Undertake continuing education and undertake roles in mammography areas such as:
  - Commissioning and acceptance testing of equipment
  - Equipment quality assurance programs
  - Radiation safety
  - Dose estimates
  - Compliance with regulatory/accreditation requirements
  - Radiation safety talks and training

Bibliography

Al Khalifah, K. H., Brindhaban, A. and Saeed, R. A. (2014). "Quality of images acquired with and without grid in digital mammo graphy." *Radiological Physics and Technology* 7(1): 109–113.

Angelone, F., Ponsiglione, A. M., Grassi, R., Amato, F. and Sansone, M. (2024). "A general framework for the assessment of scatter correction techniques in digital mammography." *Biomedical Signal Processing and Control* 89: 105802.

Davidson, R., Al Khalifah, K. and Zhou, A. (2022). "Variation in digital breast tomosynthesis image quality at differing heights above the detector." *Journal of Medical Radiation Sciences* 69(2): 174–181.

Geiser, W. R., Einstein, S. A. and Yang, W.-T. (2018). "Artifacts in digital breast tomosynthesis." *American Journal of Roentgenology* 211(4): 926–932.

Geiser, W. R., Haygood, T. M., Santiago, L., Stephens, T., Thames, D. and Whitman, G. J. (2010). "Challenges in mammography: part 1, artifacts in digital mammography." *American Journal of Roentgenology* 197: W1023–W1030.

Heggie, J. C. P., Barnes, P., Cartwright, L., Diffey, J., Tse, J., Herley, J., McLean, I. D., Thomson, F. J., Grewal, R. K. and Collins, L. T. (2017). "Position paper: recommendations for a digital mammo graphy quality assurance program V4.0." *Australasian Physical & Engineering Sciences in Medicine* 40(3): 491–543.

Logullo, A. F., Prigenzi, K. C. K., Nimir, C., Franco, A. F. V. and Campos, M. (2022). "Breast microcalcifications: past, present and future (Review)." *Molecular and Clinical Oncology* 16(4): 81.

Maki, A. K., Mainprize, J. G. and Yaffe, M. J. (2016). "Technical note: robust measurement of the slice-sensitivity profile in breast tomosynthesis." *Medical Physics* 43(8 Part1): 4803–4807.

NCRP (1988). Quality assurance for diagnostic imaging equipment. *NCRP report; no.99*. Bethesda, Md, National Council on Radiation Protection and Measurements.

Tirada, N., Li, G., Dreizin, D., Robinson, L., Khorjekar, G., Dromi, S. and Ernst, T. (2019). "Digital breast tomosynthesis: physics, artifacts, and quality control considerations." *RadioGraphics* 39(2): 413–426.

Tsalafoutas, I. A., Epistatou, A. C. and Delibasis, K. K. (2022). "Image quality comparison between digital breast tomosynthesis images and 2D mammographic images using the CDMAM test object." *Journal of Imaging* 8(8).

Vrbaski, S., Peña, L. M. A., Brombal, L., Donato, S., Taibi, A., Contillo, A. and Longo, R. (2023). "Characterization of breast tissues in density and effective atomic number basis via spectral X-ray computed tomography." *Physics in Medicine and Biology* 68.

7 Artificial Intelligence in Mammography

Chapter at a Glance

- Introduction to Artificial Intelligence
- Computer Vision in Medical Imaging
- Image Enhancement
- Segmentation
- Object Classification
- Diagnosis
- Conclusions
- Bibliography

Introduction to Artificial Intelligence

Artificial intelligence (AI) is seen almost everywhere when using computers that are online and connected to the internet. AI has many applications, and these are growing. It is now a recognized method of undertaking online searches, providing information (although the accuracy of the information should be checked) and aiding in undertaking complex computer tasks, and has applications in medical imaging.

Digital Mammography: Physics and Instrumentation, Second Edition.
Rob Davidson.
© 2026 John Wiley & Sons Ltd. Published 2026 by John Wiley & Sons Ltd.

Below is an example of an AI application in providing information.

Note: *The section below was created by Microsoft Copilot, a generative AI program. Microsoft Copilot was used via the University of Canberra's licensed Microsoft agreement under the author's UC login to provide an example of writing using artificial intelligence. The question prompt to MS Copilot was* "create a 1000 word introduction to the use of convolutional neural networks and deep learning in artificial intelligence with applications in computer vision and medical imaging."

Introduction to Convolutional Neural Networks and Deep Learning in Artificial Intelligence

Convolutional neural networks (CNNs) and deep learning have revolutionized the field of artificial intelligence (AI), particularly in applications related to computer vision and medical imaging. While I (*Microsoft Copilot*) can't provide a full essay here, I can certainly give you a comprehensive overview to get you started.

What are Convolutional Neural Networks?

Convolutional neural networks (CNNs) are a class of deep neural networks specifically designed for processing structured grid data, such as images. They are inspired by the visual cortex of animals and are particularly effective in recognizing patterns and structures in visual data. CNNs consist of multiple layers, including convolutional layers, pooling layers, and fully connected layers, each playing a unique role in feature extraction and classification.

The Role of Deep Learning

Deep learning is a subset of machine learning that involves neural networks with many layers (hence "deep"). These networks can automatically learn and extract features from raw data, making them highly effective for complex tasks such as image and speech recognition, natural language processing, and more. Deep learning models, including CNNs, have achieved state-of-the-art performance in various domains due to their ability to learn hierarchical representations of data.

Applications in Computer Vision

Image Classification

One of the primary applications of CNNs in computer vision is image classification. CNNs can be trained to recognize and categorize objects within images. For example, they can distinguish between different types of animals, vehicles, or even handwritten digits. This capability is fundamental to many AI applications, from autonomous vehicles to facial recognition systems.

Object Detection

Beyond classification, CNNs are also used for object detection, which involves identifying and localizing objects within an image. Techniques such as Region-based CNN (R-CNN) and its variants (Fast R-CNN, Faster R-CNN) have been developed to improve the speed and accuracy of object detection. These models are crucial for applications like surveillance, robotics, and augmented reality.

Image Segmentation

Image segmentation is another critical application where CNNs excel. This task involves partitioning an image into segments or regions, each representing a different object or part of an object. Semantic segmentation assigns a class label to each pixel, while instance segmentation distinguishes between different instances of the same object class. Applications include medical imaging, autonomous driving, and scene understanding.

Applications in Medical Imaging

Disease Diagnosis

CNNs have shown great promise in medical imaging, particularly in disease diagnosis. For instance, CNNs can analyze medical images such as x-rays, MRIs, and CT scans to detect abnormalities and diseases like cancer, pneumonia, and diabetic retinopathy. These models can assist radiologists by providing a second opinion and highlighting areas of concern, potentially leading to earlier and more accurate diagnoses.

Image Reconstruction

In medical imaging, obtaining high-quality images is crucial for accurate diagnosis. CNNs are used in image reconstruction to enhance the quality of medical images. For example, they can improve the resolution of MRI scans or reduce noise in CT images, making it easier for healthcare professionals to interpret the results.

Personalized Medicine

Deep learning models, including CNNs, are also being used to develop personalized medicine approaches. By analyzing medical images and patient data, these models can help tailor treatments to individual patients based on their unique characteristics. This can lead to more effective and targeted therapies, improving patient outcomes.

Conclusion

Convolutional neural networks and deep learning have transformed the landscape of artificial intelligence, particularly in the fields of computer vision and medical imaging. Their ability to automatically learn and extract features from complex data has led to significant advancements in image classification, object detection, image segmentation, disease diagnosis, image reconstruction, and personalized medicine. As research and technology continue to evolve, we can expect even more innovative applications and improvements in these areas, ultimately enhancing our ability to understand and interact with the world around us.

Note: The above section was created by Microsoft Copilot, a generative AI program. It was used under the license of the author. The purpose of the above was to both provide an example of AI information searching and writing and to also provide some background information of AI in medical imaging.

Computer Vision in Medical Imaging

Computer-based imaging has been available in medical imaging for many decades. As discussed in Chapter 3, mammography was the last medical imaging modality to fully embrace digital image capture and display. However, now that mammography has become fully digital, mammography image display and interpretation can take advantage of the latest and growing computer vision technology.

Once a medical image is captured, computer-based processes can be undertaken. In mammographic imaging, the broad categories are the same as for all medical imaging and the processes are:

- image enhancement
- segmentation and object detection
- object classification
- diagnosis

Image Enhancement

Image enhancement in mammography is briefly discussed in Chapter 3. The purpose of image enhancement is to:

- reduce noise
- enhance image contrast
- enhance spatial detail

with the purpose of enhancing the ability of viewers and AI processes to detect objects.

These processes can be manually applied by the image viewer or computer-based. CNNs, briefly discussed above by MS Copilot, are a method within AI and can be used in image enhancement. An example is noise reduction. The main form of noise in mammography is scatter radiation and CNN processes have been shown to reduce the amount of scatter visualized in the image.

Segmentation

Segmentation is the process of dividing or partitioning segments of the image into sub-regions or regions and then grouping these into objects. There are many methods of segmentation, and these include:

- Thresholding: A process of grouping pixels based on their values, either above or below the value threshold or within a range of pixel values.

- Edge-based segmentation: A digital image process of finding the edge of an object which can aid in determining the size and shape of the object.
- Region-based segmentation: A method of grouping pixels, based on predefined criteria such as intensity or texture, into objects.
- Watershed segmentation: A method that treats the image as a topographic surface and finds the lines that separate different regions based on the gradient, the value, and the distance apart of the pixels, of the image.
- Clustering-based segmentation: This uses a method by pixel statistics such as the Gaussian distribution of the values, for example, using the Gaussian Mixture Models (GMM) approach or using distance and direction of the pixel distribution, for example, using the k-means clustering method.
- Deep learning-based segmentation: Various methods of using CNN approaches, which incorporate many methods such as those above.

Object Classification

The classification of objects, that is naming and describing an object in the image, is a rapidly improving field and is primarily due to the advancement in AI methods. There are several types of object classification, and these include computer-aided detection (CADe) and radiomics. While formally there are differences between the two, they both involve in identifying objects in the image. The main differences are:

- CADe systems are designed to assist radiologists and interpreting clinicians by automatically detecting and highlighting potential abnormalities in medical images.

■ radiomics focuses on extracting and analyzing objects in the images and then quantifying the features of the objects to aid in determining what the object is. For example, features that are described by radiomic methods can be used to differentiate between benign and malignant lesions. Studies have shown that radiomic analysis can identify subtle differences in texture, shape, and intensity that are not visible to the human observer.

Object classification methods do however have several challenges. One of the main issues is the need for large, high-quality datasets of known objects for training and validation. Acquiring, and accurately describing and validating objects in these datasets is needed. The same object, for example a ductal carcinoma in the breast, can have many and varied image features that come not only from the cancer itself but also from the imaging protocols, equipment, and patient populations.

Diagnosis

The broad term for nonhuman diagnosis of medical imaging is computer-aided diagnosis (CADx). CADx now involves the use of AI, which is a broad term itself. AI encompasses the processes of deep learning. Deep learning goes beyond what was called machine learning and was an earlier CADx process. Machine learning uses computer-based algorithms such as decision trees and linear regression to extract knowledge of objects from known object data.Deep learning uses artificial neural networks (ANNs) to learn from data. The structure of the ANN is called a convolutional neural network (CNN). The process in these neural networks operates similarly to the process of the brain, hence the use of the term neural.

AI/deep learning CADx methods are growing in value in mammography diagnosis. The main reasons are

■ Improved accuracy over previous CADx methods: AI algo-rithms, particularly deep learning methods, can analyze mammograms with high precision, reducing the chances of false positives and false negatives, that is, providing a more accurate diagnosis.

■ Efficiency: AI systems can rapidly process large volumes of all types of breast images such as mammogram, contrast-enhanced mammography, digital breast tomosynthesis, MRI, and ultrasound. This assists radiologists and inter-preting clinicians by prioritizing cases that need immediate attention and highlighting areas in the image of concern.

■ Support for radiologists and interpreting clinicians: Many countries, especially in screening mammography pro-grams where the majority of examinations are negative, require all mammography examinations to be double-read to improve diagnostic accuracy. The use of AI to replace one of the interpreting clinicians is currently being evaluated in many countries.

■ Consistency: Human performance of reading mammo-graphy images, as in all things, can vary depending on fatigue and other human-related issues. Computer-based AI does not have these issues.

■ Predictive capabilities: A current trend within AI is to evaluate image features so as to predict the likelihood of malignancy and assess the risk of breast cancer and recurrence in women who have previously had a dia-gnosis of breast cancer.

Conclusions

Image enhancement and the diagnosis of breast conditions, especially malignant breast cancers, are continually being improved and AI lead approaches are the current focus. There is debate about whether AI can replace humans in making a diagnosis in many areas of medical imaging, including mammography. To me, AI in making a diagnosis is a complementary approach similar to medical imaging modalities where there are complementary modalities, and these modalities have not disappeared. For example, CT, MRI, and ultrasound did not replace planar X-ray when they were developed, and SPECT and PET have not replaced CT, MRI, and ultrasound. AI should and will complement and enhance the abilities of radiologists and interpreting clinicians and should not replace them.

Bibliography

Abdelhafiz, D., Yang, C., Ammar, R. and Nabavi, S. (2019). "Deep convolutional neural networks for mammography: advances, challenges and applications." *BMC Bioinformatics* 20(11): 281.

Avanzo, M., Stancanello, J., Pirrone, G., Drigo, A. and Retico, A. (2024). "The evolution of artificial intelligence in medical imaging: from computer science to machine and deep learning." *Cancers* 16(21): 3702.

Bahl, M. (2020). "Artificial intelligence: a Primer for breast imaging radiologists." *Journal of Breast Imaging* 2(4): 304–314.

Gillies, R. J., Kinahan, P. E. and Hricak, H. (2016). "Radiomics: images are more than pictures, they are data." *Radiology* 278(2): 563–577.

Haneberg, A. G., Pierre, K., Winter-Reinhold, E., Hochhegger, B., Peters, K. R., Grajo, J., Arreola, M., Asadizanjani, N., Bian, J., Mancuso, A. and Forghani, R. (2023). "Introduction to radiomics and artificial intelligence: a Primer for radiologists." *Seminars in Roentgenology* 58(2): 152–157.

Hosny, A., Parmar, C., Quackenbush, J., Schwartz, L. H. and Aerts, H. J. W. L. (2018). "Artificial intelligence in radiology." *Nature Reviews Cancer* 18(8): 500–510.

Mahmood, T., Li, J., Pei, Y., Akhtar, F., Rehman, M. U. and Wasti, S. H. (2022). "Breast lesions classifications of mammographic images using a deep convolutional neural network-based approach." *PLoS One* 17(1): e0263126.

Saini, V., Khurana, M. and Challa, R. K. (2025). VGG-inspired convolutional neural network denoiser for the enhancement of mammogram images. *Machine Learning Algorithms*. Cham, Springer Nature Switzerland.

Salama, W. M. and Aly, M. H. (2021). "Deep learning in mammography images segmentation and classification: automated CNN approach." *Alexandria Engineering Journal* 60(5): 4701–4709.

Seeram, E. and Kanade, V. (2024). *Artificial Intelligence in Medical Imaging Technology: An Introduction*. Springer Nature Switzerland, Cham.

Shimokawa, D., Takahashi, K., Oba, K., Takaya, E., Usuzaki, T., Kadowaki, M., Kawaguchi, K., Adachi, M., Kaneno, T., Fukuda, T., Yagishita, K., Tsunoda, H. and Ueda, T. (2023). "Deep learning model for predicting the presence of stromal invasion of breast cancer on digital breast tomosynthesis." *Radiological Physics and Technology* 16(3): 406–413.

Suzuki, Y., Hanaoka, S., Tanabe, M., Yoshikawa, T. and Seto, Y. (2023). "Predicting breast cancer risk using radiomics features of mammography images." *Journal of Personalized Medicine* 13(11): 1528.

Tang, X. (2019). "The role of artificial intelligence in medical imaging research." *BJR|Open* 2(1).

Taylor, C. R., Monga, N., Johnson, C., Hawley, J. R. and Patel, M. (2023). "Artificial intelligence applications in breast imaging: current status and future directions." *Diagnostics (Basel)* 13(12).

Index

Digital Mammography: Physics and Instrumentation, Second Edition.
Rob Davidson.
© 2026 John Wiley & Sons Ltd. Published 2026 by John Wiley & Sons Ltd.